# THE
# Love
# DIET

# THE Love DIET

## Juan-Carlos Cruz & Amy Reiley

life of reiley

*To Jennifer and Seth*
*for their undying dedication to field research.*

ISBN: 0-9774120-3-2
san 2 5 7 – 5 1 2 4
designer: Deborah Daly
creative editor: Ronie Reiley
copy editor: Mark Siagh
editorial assistants: Delahna Flagg, Sarah Goss
illustrations: Kersti Frigell
photography: Margeaux Bestard
photo stylist: Courtney Cady
recipe testers: Larisa A. Buch; Carol Stager Commons; Debbie Dillard; Ngoc Hoang; Rita & Mike Kassak; Laura & Jason Malartsik; Jenifer Marom; Kellee Mendoza; Marie Mercier; Rich Pedine; Paula Peterson; Jessica Rabbiner; Kendra Schussel; Jill Sazama; Nancy Siegel; Shane Soldinger; Nicolette Teo

Published by Life of Reiley, www.lifeofreiley.com

# Contents

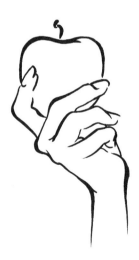

*Introduction*

# What is
# The Love Diet?

We would like to get one thing straight right off the bat: The focus of this book is not a quick trip to a bikini body. What The Love Diet offers is a road map to a delicious, balanced life packed with ingredients beneficial to sexual health. You will probably notice improved mood, more energy and you may even experience improved sleep habits as a result of your new eating plan—oh, and did we mention you will also be eating modern, sexy, interesting and tasty food from fast and easy recipes?

What is unique about the love diet is that, unlike most healthy eating plans, we bring our diet to you from a culinary perspective. In other words, TASTE (not calories, not nutrients, not fads nor peer pressure) is the deciding factor for what we choose to put in our mouths! We've both cooked for a living. We love food.

And unlike the authors of most diet books, we're committed to flavor as much as to a balanced diet.

We are also uniquely qualified to share with you our plan for a road map to sexual, sensual health through food. We've both struggled with the kind of problems addressed in this book. And we've both been able to overcome our health issues through food.

## Juan-Carlos' Story

Like most chefs, I am a complete sensualist. But with that love of sensations comes a penchant for bad habits. Most chefs smoke (which always catches me by surprise since smoking is well known to deaden sense of taste and smell). We also drink way too much. Moderation is not something chefs do well. But I never consciously related with the bad boys. In fact, when I read Anthony Bourdain's *Kitchen Confidential,* I said to my wife Jennifer, "I'm not like these pirates that drink, smoke and chase waitresses around the kitchen! I don't smoke, I certainly don't drink to excess and I've been with the same woman for 33 years. I guess that makes me the exception to the rule." At which point she laughed and told me, "You do full-contact marital arts with folks half your age. You travel around Los Angeles on a Harley and you have been inventively seducing the same woman for 33 years. You just chase sensations in your own way."

One sensation I most definitely fell victim to was the exciting tastes and textures of food; in fact, I call myself a recovering pastry chef. I've always loved cooking and although I got my full chef's degree, it was my fondness for sweets that steered my career. Years of working as a pastry chef packed on the pounds. I started cooking school at about 180 pounds and topped out at around 280.

At my heaviest, my gallbladder spoke out in protest. And, inevitably, my doctor gave me the news, "LOSE WEIGHT NOW!" The very same day the doc laid down the law, I learned that I'd been cast on a reality weight loss show for the Discovery Channel. Whatever your belief (god, karma, fate, the universe talking to you), if you don't take that kind of opportunity you are a moron!

To make a long story short, I lost a bunch of weight and even got two shows on the Food Network featuring my retooled physique and the foods that got me back to a healthy BMI. But make no mistake, anyone who tells you losing weight is easy is full of crap. Nobody gets fat overnight and you're not going to take the weight off overnight either. Doing it right is a long and steady process.

Now, I may have been losing weight for my gallbladder, but the weight loss gave me an additional, unexpected gift that has helped me stay on track for life. You see, I've made love as a fat man, skinny man and all the stages in-between and had a good time every time. But, stripped down to the basics, the male body is a hydraulic mechanism. And I must say, the more fit I am the better the quality of erection.

At my heaviest I was starting to think, "Maybe I will

*Introduction*

check into those blue pills." However, just dropping 10 pounds changed everything! When a guy loses weight, the fat pad at the base of the penis goes down. Hell, it looks like you've gained an inch or more! That alone, for me, is enough inspiration for a lifetime of exercise and eating right.

## Amy's Story

For almost 10 years, I struggled with a problem that was pretty much the polar opposite to Juan-Carlos. When I was in college, my mysterious weight loss began. I stand 5'9" and at one point, I weighed in at 89 pounds. It seemed like all anyone in my life wanted to say to me was "eat!" But I never had an appetite. I tried adding big calories in small doses, like flax seed oil in my oatmeal or protein powder in my drink. But high-fat foods often had me doubled over in pain and rich meat dishes served at the dinners I was required to attend for my job as a food writer were impossible to digest. (I've probably insulted more celebrity chefs than I can count on both hands.) My energy was low, I had no body fat to keep me warm and as for a libido? That was nonexistent.

Finally, I found a brilliant doctor, Murray Susser, who was able to help me make sense of it all, and, after about two years of trial and error with visits to nutritionists, digestive supplements regimes and exams of every kind, Dr. Susser and I struck upon the formula for gain. It turns out, all the antibiotics I was fed as a kid for chronic sinus infections had given me a systemic yeast infection that went undiagnosed for years. As a result, I wound up with very little stomach acid. Here I was, a woman who loved food so much I made it my profession, and I couldn't digest it!

Among his treatments, Dr. Susser put me on vitamin C and amino acid IV's. I had already delved into the world of aphrodisiacs at this point in my career and was fascinated by the nutritional aspect of aphrodisiac foods. So a treatment for my weight issue based on heavy-duty vitamin therapy sparked my interest in learning everything I could about the nutritional side of aphrodisiacs.

Sadly, shortly after I began a successful recovery (about 10 pounds in five months), Dr. Susser retired. But his successor, Dr. Allen Green (who I still see today), suggested completing my treatment by supplementing my sluggish thyroid. (I was probably the skinniest person in history with a hypothyroid.) The medication was miraculous and for the first time in years, I had an appetite. Suddenly, I was eating twice as much as I had at any point in my adult life and digesting it!

But I still had one side effect of my illness to treat: my libido. This one, I knew, I could handle on my own. I started applying all the information I had been gathering on libido-boosting foods. These ingredients, coupled with a desire for romance and a passion for the sensual pleasures of food, had me on track in no time. Before I knew it, I was playing around with nutrient-rich recipes as the vehicle for my first book, *Fork Me, Spoon Me.*

When people ask me if aphrodisiacs really work, here is what I tell them: While I was testing recipes for the book, my roommate introduced me to a friend of hers who was the consummate bachelor. We'll call him Mr. Takeout. Because I was cooking every day, I would invite Mr. Takeout over to sample the dishes, figuring I'd save him a few delivery charges. Eventually, *Fork Me, Spoon Me,* along with my recovery, was finished and Mr. Takeout was still around. Today we share a life, a home and many, many romantic meals.

### This is Not a Quick Fix!

The Love Diet is not a short-term fix like a grapefruit diet or a fat flush. What we are offering you are building blocks for eating interesting, tasty, sensory-awakening foods now and forever, for a lifetime of health (and some serious stamina in the bedroom!).

# 1
# Getting with the Program
## *how to use this book*

Let's face it, every body is different and we all have different wants and desires (in the kitchen and in the bedroom). Like your wardrobe or your taste in lovers, your Love Diet should be personal. To help you decide what it is you want, we've divided the recipes into chapters based on their amorous effects. But don't think you should just find "your" section and stick to it. That would be a gastronomic snore. Because all the recipes in this book incorporate ingredients to give your lifestyle a healthy kick in the pants and your body a "lift" in the bedroom, you can definitely mix it up between the chapters (and between the sheets).

Now, we're not going to present you with a regimented day-by-day eating plan—neither of us could stick to that, so why should we expect it of you? What The Love Diet does is introduces you to simple, taste bud tickling, sexy recipes packed with nutrients beneficial for sexual health. What we recommend is that you focus on the recipe chapter that best meets your goal right now, incorporating recipes from other sections as they best fit with your lifestyle. (We know that your goal will probably change in time and your favorite chapter should definitely change with you.)

To begin, for example, you may make a plan with Cook Me Sexy (lower calorie foods) but two or three days per week cook up Quickies as an alternative to fast food. And then once or twice a month schedule a Romantic Weekend with more indulgent dishes that you can cook together (or that you can sit back and watch him or her cook, wearing nothing more than an apron).

## Leftovers Can Be Sexy

We've designed most of the recipes in this book to make four servings. Yes, the idea of our book is recipes for you and a partner. But frankly, we love our leftovers.

We look at designing recipes for four as giving you the gift of a day without cooking for every day you put in your time in the kitchen. (Not to mention that our emotions are very easily triggered by the senses and often the scent of leftovers can reignite the passion the dish sparked when it was first served.) Sometimes, you may find yourself utterly famished from the "under-the-covers tango" and eat more than two of a recipe's four servings but whatever amount is left, we hope you'll save the leftovers, perhaps packing your lover a "thanks for the memories" lunch the next day (unless you went back for seconds with a lust-charged midnight snack!).

## Singles, Couples, Families—This Book is for Everyone

This book is not just for couples. If you're single, there's no time like the present to get on the program—think how far ahead you'll be when you find Mr./Ms. Right. (In the meantime, there's more food for you!)

You can also cook from this book for your family. A friend who tried some of our recipes says the soybean dip is about the only green thing her kids will eat. And just because they're eating Love Diet foods does not automatically turn your children into wild rabbits in heat. Mother Nature takes care of that.

## Leaf Eaters on the Love Diet (Even Vegan)

You don't need meat (the kind you cook) to live on The Love Diet. We're not saying protein isn't important. In fact, studies have shown that protein can increase norepinephrine production—a neurotransmitter known as a sex booster and mood enhancer. But you'll find, as you flip through the chapters, that many of our recipes use plant-based proteins instead of meat. You may love you some beef, but trust us, rich cuts won't do much for your sex life. Think about it: What do you want to do after enjoying a big steak? Take a big nap! And frankly, we aren't particularly into supporting an industry as detrimental to the environment as the American beef biz.

So, we've tried to give you an approach to eating that still appeals to your taste buds but will have a positive impact on your figure, your love life and the planet. To further help out our vegetarian readers, we've made a special note on each recipe that's veggie-friendly. We're particularly proud to say that we even slipped in a few for the vegans. (It isn't all that common to find chefs who are down with dairy-free!)

## The Recipe Chapters

### *Boost Your Libido*

Boost your libido foods work to provide essential nutrients for boosting and/or maintaining optimal sexual health. "Aphrodisiacs" is a word that is often tossed off as being as mythological as the goddess for which they're named. But thanks to modern research, we're learning that those foods held in regard as "aphrodisiacs" by ancient cultures actually have nutritional properties that can benefit libido. In some cases, they have the potential to replace prescription medication. (And in many cases, if you start early they can help avoid the need for medical help in the under-the-covers department—for life.)

### Quickies

These are the recipes for those of us who want a fulfilling romantic life but don't really have the time to slave over the stove for sexual health. (Trust us, we don't want to waste our last bit of energy hunched over a pot, either.) Make dinner a Quickie, then use your power reserves to stir up some lust.

### Romantic Weekends

The romance recipes are our "splurge" foods. You can't eat these dishes all the time and expect to sport the figure of a supermodel. You also probably can't afford to, since this chapter also uses some of the rare and luxurious ingredients that make the heart swoon and the wallet deflate. It is our "have your cake and eat it too" chapter (and yes, there is even a chocolate cake recipe). Romantic Weekend dishes are indulgent (but within reason) and should be used only occasionally to make them seem even more special.

### Little Blue Pill Foods

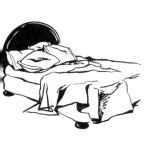

Our Little Blue Pill recipes contain ingredients that have an immediate effect on the body in readying it for the primal pas de deux. If you're on the hunt and want to plan a night of seduction, we consider these your "sure thing" foods. Using ingredients like chile, ginger and coffee that are known from nutritional science to give a surge of energy, elevate mood, raise body temperature and/or give your date a giddy moment, we offer you our best bets for one night (or day) of passion.

## Cook Me Sexy

These are our reduced calorie/cholesterol/fat versions of nutrition-packed "comfort" foods. They are easy, everyday dishes that you and your lover can cook together as you work to lose or maintain your ideal weight. But know that, while you're eating in "moderation," you're also ingesting all sorts of aphrodisiac ingredients, so you'll not only look great but feel frisky.

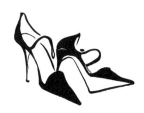

## Nibbles, Snacks and a Little Something on the Side

Not going to lie, we're snackers. And we recommend that—if you haven't already—you should join the snack tribe. Look, our mealtime recipes exercise portion control. We find it is better for sustained energy to eat three reasonable-sized meals and then fill out the day with a snack every few hours—including a bedtime snack. (After all, when do you need energy in a sexually fulfilled life? When you're in bed. And what gives you energy? Food! So don't be afraid to have a little something late at night. Play your cards right and you'll burn it off by morning.)

## Dictionary of Desire—Discovering Ingredients That Work for You

Because we realize that it simply isn't realistic to expect you to eat at home all the time, we've offered you a little additional guidance with our Dictionary of Desire. This section will help you in choosing smart snacks and can guide you toward the foods to choose when you travel or dine out. But just remember: We know how to cook, we sure know how to eat we know a heck of a lot about food but we are not doctors. So before you go drastically changing your intake of any one nutrient, run it by a medical professional.

## Stop and Smell the Stock Pot

It's plainly obvious that we live in a fast-paced world. One of the secrets to a fulfilling meal (and a fulfilling sex life) is to be present in the experience. We've created The Love Diet recipes with this important factor in mind. As you tune in to your food, you'll notice that many of our dishes have a variety of textures and temperatures (and sometimes even aromas) on one plate. We think this kind of variety really up's the sensuality of a meal by engaging and challenging the senses.

## Don't Kid Yourself, You've Got to Get Some Exercise

The truth might hurt, but you'll never get your libido in tip-top shape without a little exercise. We are both committed to regular exercise—and not just to stay trim. Exercising regularly can give you more energy and improve your stamina (how else can you expect to perform the horizontal cha-cha to perfection?). It is

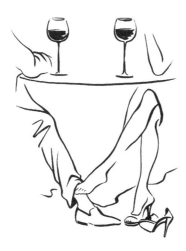

also wonderful for stress reduction and general relaxation (both of which will be reflected in your performance in the bedroom).

The trick is to find the form of exercise that turns you on—and it doesn't have to involve a gym. Amy is addicted to the Wii and will spend hours on the Fit Board. Juan-Carlos signs up for full-contact martial arts several nights each week. But if you really hate exercise in every guise, then at the very least take advantage of your weekly chores as workout time. Park in the very last row at the grocery store then trade in the wheeled cart for a hand-held basket. (Try squatting to reach for a few cans on bottom shelves with a gallon of milk in your basket and you'll have some fine looking quads in no time.)

Oh, and P.S. Smoking, lack of sleep and vending machines are leading killers of your sex life.

# 2
# The Love Diet Pantry

*foods to have on hand, ingredients to grow and tools to deck out your kitchen*

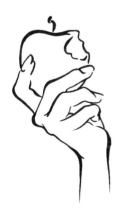

As you read through our recipes, you'll notice that we don't believe in banning foods. Our kitchens are stocked with butter, a variety of oils, sugar, salt, bacon, mayo, vodka and just about every other diet taboo. We just employ these ingredients judiciously, using just enough to deliver the desired flavor. Then we round out the recipes with other natural ingredients that add layers of complexity and provide ultimate satisfaction (in the dining room and beyond).

What's going to make embarking on The Love Diet easy is a little pantry makeover.  We're not going to come in and rip all the packages of instant chocolate pudding from your clutches. But we are going to advise you on some items you should add to your arsenal to help make cooking from this book a pleasure. (And if you started to squirm at the mention of a pantry makeover, you should probably also put some serious thought into foods you might want to 86. No judgment here, but in our experience, a guilty conscious usually equates to some serious crap in the cupboards.)

## Spice it Up

The best place to start is your spice rack. Variety of spices is, well, the spice of life! Spices are also a huge part of The Love Diet. Historically, spices have been used since the beginning of recorded time as potent aphrodisiacs. And from a culinary standpoint, they add flavor without unnecessary fat, for which we love them doubly much.

But keep in mind that spices do not last forever. We give them about a six-month lifespan. Write the date on the spice jar when you purchase it to keep track of its expiration. Then dump when you notice it's overdue. You can also try lengthening your spices' shelf lives with the prepackaged spice grinders that have suddenly become so popular. (Whole spices last longer than those that have been pre-ground.) This packaging allows you to grind the spice yourself at the moment you use it for the greatest flavor impact.

Some of the spices you will find on our shelves include:

### chile powder

Even if, like Amy, you're a little bit shy of heat, chile powder is a MUST for every smart and sexy kitchen. Used in small doses, it is one of the world's most effective aphrodisiacs because of its ability to raise body temperature and heart rate, as well as make the tongue tingle. Best of all, studies have shown chiles to help speed metabolism, (naysayers maintain the effects are probably negligible—but we're all for the power of positive thinking!).

### whole, dried chile peppers

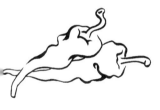

We love dried chiles for the same reasons we recommend chile powder, however as a flavoring agent, whole peppers can offer much more variety than a generic ground spice. Some of our favorite chiles for bringing complexity of flavor to casseroles, soups and stews include straightforward Anchos, smoky Chipotles and daringly spicy Thai chiles.

### paprika

Paprika is made of powdered, mild chiles. As a result, its color is a vibrant red but its flavor delicate. Although it is a typical flavoring in Hungarian cuisine, paprika is often overlooked in American kitchens—but not The Love Diet kitchen! We use it to add mild heat and a subtle complexity to dishes that can raise body temperature without setting the tongue on fire.

*The Love Diet Pantry*

*coriander powder*

Some foods only offer flavor on the tip of the tongue, others sort of settle at the back of your mouth. A satisfying dish offers flavor across the whole palate. One of the items in the arsenal we reach for when a dish is missing a part of the mouth is ground coriander. Coriander tends to add flavor right on the center of the tongue. Used sparingly, it can make a dish more satisfying by tickling all the taste buds without much alteration to flavor.

*white and black peppercorns*

Throughout this book, we call for "freshly ground pepper." We don't use the pre-ground stuff. After it's ground, the pepper loses its dimensions of flavor (and very often its made from inferior peppercorns). White has a milder flavor than black but unless a recipe specifies either black or white, use the pepper of your preference—just so long as you grind it yourself! (And watch out, we just might come over to check.)

*cinnamon, nutmeg and allspice*

Cinnamon, the most common of the "warming spices," is probably already residing in your spice rack. But consider adding its counterparts, nutmeg and allspice, to your collection. All three were historically used as aphrodisiacs for their ability to warm the body (and the heart!). The three work similarly to add body and flavor to baked goods but the variety of flavors to choose from will keep your cooking from growing mundane.

*whole cloves*

Like the aforementioned spices, cloves work to raise body temperature. They are most commonly sold as a ground spice but we love adding whole cloves to a pot of steaming rice, poached fruit or even tea to add a faintly spicy note without the serious heat of a chile. Use them as you would a bay leaf and be sure to remove them before serving.

*sea salt*

Salt is not the enemy. The sodium in processed foods is an enemy. But a nice, natural salt can bring vibrancy to a dish without harm to your body—we need salt to keep our electrolytes in balance. And when you add the salt yourself, you can cut back as needed. However, when cooking, if a recipe calls for salt in two different places, say for example, you are supposed to sauté the vegetables with salt and then finish the dish with salt to taste, we recommend reducing the salt in each step rather than omitting it entirely from one step. (This way, you'll still get the desired development of flavors but a milder, lower sodium flavor.)

We use sea salt, which contains beneficial trace minerals. As you start to cook with salt, you'll find there is a wide range of sea (and lake) salts on the market—some with lower sodium than others (check the nutrition label). We're also starting to get into all the "flavored" salts now on the market, infused with herbs, blended with cacao, citrus peel, ground nuts or even blended with truffle shavings. We encourage you to start exploring the world of salt as a part of your personal Love Diet.

## The Love Diet Refrigerator

In your refrigerator, you should always keep a number of staples. It isn't a full refrigerator that will lead you down the path to temptation, it's an empty one that's a problem. Without the tools to cook sensual meals at your fingertips, you're just one speed dial away from libido-deadening delivery of high-fat craving foods. Here are some of the foods we recommend you always keep on hand:

*milk*

Drink what you like but we recommend skim or 1% milk. (You'll find that even if you drink non-fat, you may prefer milk with fat for cooking to help give body to certain dishes.) As you flip through this book, you'll find we also use a lot of soymilk in cooking. Yes, it's more processed than cow's milk but we prefer it in certain recipes and both always keep a carton handy.

*butter*

Unless you're vegan, butter is a must! We call for unsalted in our recipes but if you prefer salted butter on your bread, you may want to keep both kinds on hand. We also keep butter-substitute spreads in our refrigerators. Amy explains, "Although it took me awhile to adjust to the taste (and, frankly, the idea), I now love putting a (non-hydrogenated) flax-based spread on my toast. It spreads smoothly, offers beneficial Omega-3's and contains less calories than butter."

### mayonnaise

There is no reason to fear mayonnaise. A thin layer on a turkey sandwich or blended with buttermilk to make a salad dressing, you just can't beat the comfort-food flavor of mayo. Do we pile gobs of it on our tuna salad or dip vegetables into it straight? No, we don't. But used wisely, mayo can be your friend. Juan-Carlos adds, "It sounds good in theory but low-fat mayo tends to use sugar to replace the taste of fat. Rather than adding unnecessary sugar to your diet, we say go full fat, just cut down the portion."

### yogurt

Your refrigerator should contain yogurt. We love it for breakfast or a bedtime snack. Plain, non-fat Greek yogurt can also be used in a pinch as a substitute for sour cream or crème fraîche (we've even served this to chefs who haven't recognized the difference).

### turkey or ham deli slices

Although it is processed and can contain a lot of sodium, lunchmeat is great to have on hand for chasing away the midday slump. It is also a good preworkout snack and can help you sustain energy during a strenuous trip to the gym. Be sure to look for products that are nitrate-free.

### cheese

Our refrigerators are almost never without a wedge of high-quality, hard cheese. An ounce of cheese offers the protein to keep the body going between meals. We like strong-flavored cheeses because a little bit goes a long way. Slice up a small wedge to top apple, celery or cucumber pieces or a handful of rye or wheat crackers. Hard cheese is also great to have on hand to add complexity to a pan of sautéed vegetables, pasta with fresh tomatoes or scrambled egg whites.

## *eggs*

A carton of eggs is almost an insta-meal at the ready, a perfect row of little soldiers poised for action on the refrigerator shelf. If you have eggs on hand, you can whip up a quick breakfast or dinner and you're always ready to bake. We usually keep both eggs and egg beaters in the fridge because although we love eggs, we also enjoy the variety.

## *flax seed oil*

If you've ever heard the recommendation to eat oily fish regularly or take fish oil capsules but are turned off by the fishy taste, flax seed oil is the ingredient for you. Made from those tiny, brown seeds found in many European breads, flax seed oil, like fish oil, contains those beneficial Omega-3 fatty acids but without the taste of fish. Use it as a healthy topping for salad greens, sautéed spinach or any vegetable dish. Amy also likes a teaspoon of the oil on top of her oatmeal. Always apply flax seed oil after the dish is cooked. Cooking with the oil will destroy many of its beneficial properties.

## *lemons*

No refrigerator should be without this most versatile

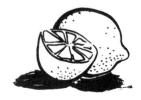

citrus. Lemons add a burst of flavor to your dish without unnecessary calories and fat. We love using lemon juice and zest in everything from marinades to salad dressings to desserts.

### ginger

Fresh ginger root is an inexpensive, low-cal flavoring with a lot of impact. Better yet, ginger will not only heighten flavor, it also raises body temperature and can increase adrenalin, both proven to kick in those primal urges.

### colorful, ripe fruits and vegetables

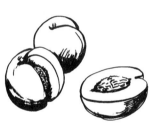

This one may be common sense, but we find that keeping a bowl of fruits and vegetables on the counter or at eye level in the refrigerator keeps us reaching for the good stuff instead of culinary junk. The trick is to stock the fruit bowl with beautiful, fresh produce at least twice a week, making sure to pick items in a variety of colors. Some of our favorites, depending on the season, include: blueberries; raspberries; strawberries; peaches; figs; cherries; mangos; pineapple; watermelon; carrots; cucumbers; spring onions; celery; tomatoes; arugula and avocado.

### Champagne

A Love Diet house is not a home without bubbly at the ready! All too many of us think of sparkling wine as only a special occasion drink, but with a bottle always available, you're ready to turn any day into a special day. (Not only a giddy drink to get the guard down, Champagne has the antioxidant benefits of red wine and some beneficial nutrients for brain health.)

## In the Love Diet Cupboards

### *white and whole wheat flour*

We recommend keeping both kinds of flour on hand. We're not going to tell you to banish all white things on this diet. But we do like to mix up the white with the whole grain, which will add nutritional *umph* to your diet.

### *dark chocolate*

No Love Diet kitchen should ever be without sexifying, premium dark chocolate. A good dark chocolate makes an incredibly gratifying snack with the bonus of antioxidants. It also has many uses in cooking both savory and sweet dishes and can be finely chopped and tossed into warm milk for a sultry bedtime snack.

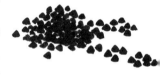

### *garlic*

Yes, its true that both members of a couple must indulge in garlic together if the meal's ultimate goal is a make out session but when you consider garlic's health benefits, why wouldn't you? Garlic is credited with fighting everything from colds to cancer—more importantly for the aspiring lover—it raises body temperature and boosts stamina. When you're choosing garlic at the store, look for bulbs with tight skin. The garlic should feel firm when squeezed. Any green shoots coming out of the top indicate an old bulb, which should be discarded. (We both cop to having jars of preminced garlic at the ready. Its flavor lacks the depth of fresh garlic, but for times when convenience outweighs complexity of flavor, we both reach for the jar. It's not a crime.)

## yellow onion, sweet onion and shallots

Onions lend a dish so much flavor, we don't dare ever let our kitchens run out. Most cooks keep brown onions around, which are delicious sautéed or sweated. But we like to keep a variety on hand, including Vidalia, those onions so sweet you can bite into them raw, as well as shallots (which are not actually onions but a close relative) for their mild flavor that hints of garlic without the bad breath.

## Dijon mustard

Until modern times, it was believed that mustard was such a potent aphrodisiac that monks weren't permitted the condiment. We particularly like the mild heat and intense flavor of Dijon, which can wake up the taste of any bland dish.

## balsamic vinegar

Like lemons, balsamic can brighten the flavor of a dish. Its sweetness and richness will also add depth. We recommend spending a couple extra dollars to buy quality vinegar but it is by no means necessary to buy the most expensive product on the shelf. (You will probably want to keep at least one more kind of vinegar in your pantry. In addition to balsamic, we both keep red wine, apple cider and rice wine vinegars. You don't necessarily need all four. As you begin to cook, you will figure out for yourself which products to stock.)

## good olive oil, cooking spray and "neutral" oils

A nice-quality olive oil is a must for your pantry. You should also have a neutral-flavored oil like grape seed. (Grape seed oil offers many of the same antioxidant benefits as red wine.) In addition, we recommend you stock your kitchen with an inexpensive vegetable oil (also considered "neutral" because it doesn't impart additional flavor to the dish), which is indispensable for baking. In many of The Love Diet recipes, we reduce the fat by skipping bottled oil and just using a non-stick cooking spray. (Just keep in mind that all oils will go rancid if kept too long, so don't go overboard buying oils right off the bat.)

## truffle oil

Sex in a bottle! Although it is more expensive than most cooking oils, truffle oil is actually a well-priced indulgence when you compare it to the price of whole truffles. Because the flavor of truffle is so intense, you can capture its earthy richness reasonably well in a dish by just using the oil. Since the scent of black truffle is very similar to that of a particular male pheromone, this is one indulgence we recommend, particularly for the ladies, as a great splurge item. (And Amy can personally endorse the aphrodisiac effectiveness of this one!)

## The Love Diet Garden

If you don't already have your own garden, now is the perfect time to start! Even if you don't have a yard (or a green thumb—yet), slap on your overalls because you can become a farmer. Just find one sunny windowsill for your own herb garden. Start with hearty plants like rosemary, mint and sage then work your way up to delicious flavorings like basil, parsley and chives.

Why do we think it's important to grow rather than buy your herbs? Gardening is not only great for the environment and great for your figure—gardening can give you a real workout—but it will bring you closer to the source of your food. And that kind of awareness only helps to accentuate the sensual pleasures of the table. In addition, if you graduate from herbs to fruits and vegetables, you'll be able to dine on produce at the peak of ripeness, when both flavor and nutrition are at their apex.

In our gardens—depending on the season—you'll find everything from lemons and almonds to tomatoes, lemongrass, fennel and arugula. If you're into ingredients that make a color splash, we recommend trying to grow edible flowers. We use nasturtium blossoms and violets in salads, candy fresh rose petals to decorate cakes, lavender to flavor teas and garlic and chive flowers to garnish soups.

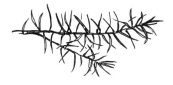

## The Culinary Tool Box

When an interest in cooking is first ignited, there's a tendency to go out and buy every tool in the store. The truth is you don't need a whole lot of equipment to be a good cook. Juan-Carlos, who has spent most of his adult life in restaurants adds, "It's fun to watch the new chefs show up to their first restaurant job with a big toolbox full of every imaginable gadget. But if you watch the old guard chefs, they bring a small, fabric knife roll with just the most necessary items."

Here are a few we recommend for making your life easy on The Love Diet:

### *knives—chef's knife, bread knife, paring knife*

Although there is a knife out there for pretty much every task, there are only two you most often need: a big chef's knife and a small paring knife. And if you like fresh bread as much as we do, you'll also want a bread knife for safely making neat slices.

### *stock pot*

The recipes in this book require very few pots and pans, but you will need to find room in your kitchen for a stockpot to use in making soups and stews.

### *small saucepan*

Since most of our recipes serve two or four, you don't need a whole stack of saucepans in different sizes. Just invest in one that is small and sturdy.

### microplane zester

This tool, based on a carpenter's rasp, isn't necessary in all kitchens but it is important for The Love Diet kitchen. It is, in our opinions, the best tool on the market for creating citrus zest—used on The Love Diet for boosting flavor without adding calories. The zester also works extremely well to finely grate small portions of cheese and chocolate.

### measuring cups and spoons

We know that some of you don't believe in detail-oriented cooking (our polite way of saying *making accurate measurements*). We fully applaud your confidence but we also believe in measuring—at least the first time we try a dish. This is particularly important with fattening ingredients like butter and oil, as well as strong ingredients like salt and chile. Get yourself a good set of dry measuring cups and spoons, as well as a liquid measuring cup.

### kitchen scale

Kitchen scales are key (and relatively inexpensive) for monitoring portion control (like double checking that that 2 oz serving of pasta isn't actually 3.5.). It will also aid in getting the most accurate measurements for things like butter, dried fruits and all the other ingredients for which too much of a good thing is simply too much.

## sturdy blender

In order to follow The Love Diet, a reliable blender is the one appliance you need. (As you get more interested in cooking, we recommend investing in a stand mixer and food processor or at least a mandolin but you really don't need these items to start.)

## immersion blender

If you aren't ready to invest in a sturdy blender, at least get yourself a small, hand-held immersion blender. Light and inexpensive, it is one of Juan-Carlos' favorite tools in the whole kitchen.

A few more inexpensive tools you'll want for cook along with us:

a good vegetable peeler; whisk; tongs and one small and one large, non-stick sauté pan.

# 3
# Boost Your Libido

This is our "eating right" starter kit. One dose of the foods in this chapter isn't going to make a remarkable difference but using these recipes as a guide to get your libido in shape is going to give you long-lasting results. Its like doing squats. One day of exercise may make your backside burn but it takes faithful lunging for a beautiful booty. You need to focus on the right ingredients every day in order to evolve that inner sex god or goddess. (For more information on the ingredients as well as more foods offering all the right stuff, visit the Dictionary of Desire, page 121.)

We think of this chapter as the starter kit for a healthy sex drive for life. (And an overall healthier you.) We're handing you the equipment. It's up to you to start basic training.

# casanova fruit smoothie

vegetarian

*makes 2 servings*

There are few ways to get a good dose of fruits and veggies before you even rub the sleep from your eyes. Because everything goes right into the blender, you can make this smoothie in about two minutes flat, get a little nutrition boost and bounce back into bed for a preshower play date.

Since you use the pear with the skin on, you're getting a nice dose of fiber, which will help prevent the blood sugar spike and crash a glass of juice can cause. Coupled with manganese-rich spinach and the scent of vanilla, this is the kind of drink with the power to turn any man into a Latin lothario.

1. Add grape juice, spinach, pear, 2 tbsp lemon juice, ginger and vanilla to blender. Purée until smooth.

2. Taste. If smoothie isn't sweet enough, add the agave nectar (it all depends on the sweetness of your pear). For additional tartness, add the last tbsp lemon juice.

3. Add ice cubes and blend on high until smooth and frothy.

4. Divide smoothie between two juice glasses to serve.

1/2 c white grape juice

1/2 c spinach

1 small, ripe bartlett or d'anjou pear (skin on), quartered and cored

2-3 tbsp lemon juice

1 tsp fresh ginger root, minced

1/4 tsp vanilla extract

1 tbsp agave nectar, (optional)

10 ice cubes

# savory watermelon salad
vegetarian

*makes 2 servings as an appetizer or side dish*

Research released in 2008 declared watermelon "nature's Viagra." What, specifically, was discovered was that one of watermelon's phytonutrients, citrulline, has the power to relax blood vessels. The body converts the citrulline to argenine and argenine boosts nitric oxide, which relaxes blood vessels (basically the same effect as Viagra—although it could take as much as 6 cups of watermelon per day to reach the desired result). Whether or not you found that explanation far too scientific, bottom line is: Eat up!

2 c watermelon (about 1lb), cut into bite-sized pieces

1 tbsp rice wine vinegar

2 tbsp fat-free feta

1/4 c Vidalia or other sweet onion, finely chopped

1/4 tsp salt

1 tbsp fresh mint, chopped

1. Toss watermelon, rice wine vinegar, feta, onion and salt in a salad bowl.

2. Gently mix in mint and serve immediately.

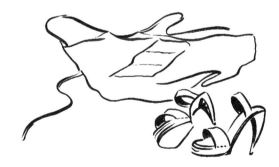

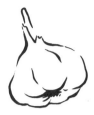

# french garlic soup
vegetarian
*makes 2–4 servings as an appetizer*

Garlic soup is an old, French cure-all. We know, it sounds crazy to center an aphrodisiac dish on garlic. But by roasting the garlic, the flavor becomes sweet, losing much of the pungence that can seep from your pores. Yet it still delivers garlic's health benefits, which, you might be surprised to learn, are many. The Ancient Greeks noted that garlic promotes energy and began feeding it to athletes prior to competition. It also offers age-defying antioxidants and may, according to recent research, even be helpful in promoting weight control.

1. Preheat oven to 400 degrees.

2. Remove any loose skin from garlic and roast, whole, in the oven for 20 minutes or until it gives slightly to the touch. Set aside until garlic is cool enough to touch.

1 head garlic, whole
4 c chicken stock
1 tsp fresh or 1/2 tsp dried thyme
salt to taste
4 fresh baguette slices
butter, (optional)

3. In a medium stockpot, bring chicken stock to a simmer.

4. When it is simmering, add in thyme. Squeeze individual garlic cloves from their skins and add to the stock.

5. Simmer for 20 minutes.

6. Pour soup into blender (or use an immersion blender) and purée until soup is smooth.

7. Return to pot and heat through before serving, seasoning with salt to taste. Serve with the baguette slices and (optional) butter.

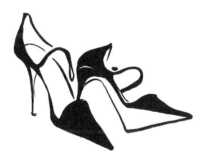

*Boost Your Libido*

# sizzling lemongrass mussels

*makes 2 servings*

Mussels rock! Easy to cook, high in protein and impressive in presentation, mussels are also a super-food for the bedroom. (One recent study discovered that an amino acid in mussels directly raised sexual hormone levels.) You are going to love this dish for all those reasons not to mention the huge impact of flavors you'll develop without even breaking a sweat. (No, really—this dish takes about 10 minutes, start-to-finish.)

1. Rinse the mussels well in cold water, discarding any that won't snap shut when handled. If the mussels have not been debearded, remove the patch of seaweed, or "beard," sticking out from between the two shells.

2. Cut the lemongrass stalks on the diagonal into 2–3 inch lengths. Using the back of a heavy kitchen knife, lightly crush the lengths of lemongrass to release the flavors.

3. In a nonstick sauté pan or wok, heat the vegetable oil over medium-high heat.

4. Sauté the shallots in the oil until edges brown, about 1 minute.

5. Add lemongrass and toss until heated through, about another minute.

6. Add the wine, chicken stock, sriracha and fish sauce (but don't smell the fish sauce—just trust us on that).

1 lb mussels
2 lemongrass stalks
2 tbsp vegetable oil
1 shallot, thinly sliced
1/2 c white wine
1/2 c chicken stock
1 tsp sriracha, (hot chili sauce)
2 tbsp fish sauce
2 tbsp cilantro leaves, coarsely chopped
2 c cooked white rice, (optional)

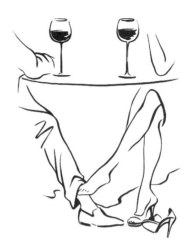

7. Bring liquid to a boil and boil for 1 minute.

8. Add the mussels, reducing heat slightly, cover and cook until all the mussels are open, about 4–5 minutes. (They may open sooner.) Remove from heat immediately and toss in cilantro.

9. Divide mussels between 2 bowls either on their own or over white rice.

# seared scallop & apple salad with a sweet potato-shallot purée

*makes 2 servings*

Yes, this recipe takes several steps to complete but don't doubt for one minute that the sweat equity isn't worth it. The layers of flavor and aphrodisiac ingredients in the final dish will have anyone fooled into thinking they're indulging in a decadent, restaurant-created feast.

*for the potatoes:*

1. Preheat the oven to 375 degrees.

2. In a shallow baking dish coated with non-stick spray, toss the sweet potatoes, cauliflower and shallots with the oil and salt.

3. Bake covered for 15 minutes. Uncover and bake for an additional 15 minutes or until potatoes are fork-tender.

4. Transfer vegetables to a blender or food processor and add 2 tbsp of milk. Purée until mixture is smooth, adding additional milk 1 tablespoon at a time until puree reaches desired consistency. Season with salt to taste.

5. Serve immediately or reheat before serving.

2 medium sweet potatoes (skins on), trimmed and cut into 1-inch pieces

1 1/2 c frozen cauliflower

2 small shallots, peeled and trimmed

1 1/2 tsp grape seed or other neutral oil

1 tsp salt

3-5 tbsp skim milk

salt to taste

2 tsp unsalted butter

1 medium Fuji or other crisp apple

8 large, wild sea scallops

pinch salt

1/4 c red wine vinegar

1 tbsp Dijon mustard

2 c baby arugula

*Note:* The puree actually makes 4 servings. Its a versatile, healthy potato dish, so we love having extra on hand for those nights when we're too busy to cook.

*for the scallops:*

1. Over medium heat, melt 1 tsp of the butter in a nonstick pan.

2. When butter is hot (but not brown), add the apples and sauté until fruit browns slightly and just begins to soften. Remove apples from pan and set aside.

3. Add the second tsp of butter and allow it to melt before returning the pan to the heat.

4. Sprinkle scallops with the pinch of salt. Add scallops to hot pan and cook until golden brown on both sides, turning once (about 3–4 minutes per side, depending on thickness of scallops).

5. Remove scallops from pan.

6. Immediately deglaze pan with the vinegar, scraping off all the cooked bits at the bottom. Remove pan from heat and stir in Dijon mustard to make a vinaigrette.

*to assemble:*

1. Divide 1/2 of the sweet potato purée between two plates. (Save the other half of the sweet potato puree to serve with grilled chicken, pork chops or your other favorite meat.)

*Boost Your Libido*

2. Top each plate with 1 cup arugula.

3. Divide apple slices and scallops between plates then drizzle with the warm dressing.

A super-sensual recipe like this deserves an equally aphrodisiac drink. We recommend a splash of vino. Because you have a combination of both hearty and delicate flavors on one plate, the dish welcomes many styles of wine. We like it with Sauvignon Blanc, Brut Sparkling Wine, Chardonnay, Pinot Noir and Syrah.

# chocolate-kissed white bean chili
vegetarian
*makes 4–6 servings*

There is a long Mexican culinary history of using chocolate in savory dishes. But we can't accurately call our creation Mexican, nor is it particularly American. What it is, is an aphrodisiac. By layering a modest dose of chile pepper with both antioxidant-rich cocoa and bittersweet chocolate, we've given the chili a surprisingly earthy base. On top of that, we've added acai, the super-fruit of the Amazon, which brings not only a powerful hit of nutrients but offers a subtle sweetness to the final flavor. All too often we've found a big bowl of chili leaves us longing for a nap. So we've omitted meat from the recipe to keep the chili light. We like to think of our chili as an invigorating parade of tastes and spices that will send you marching straight for the bedroom.

2 tbsp vegetable oil

1 small yellow onion, chopped

2 stalks celery, chopped

1 clove garlic, finely minced

12 oz soy ground meat substitute*

2 tsp-1 tbsp chile powder

1 tsp ground cumin

1/2 tsp powdered cayenne pepper

1 16 oz can diced tomatoes

1 16 oz can white beans

1 c vegetable broth

1/4 tsp dried oregano

1 bay leaf

1/4 c pure açai juice or fruit purée, (optional)**

1 oz bittersweet chocolate, grated (or chocolate chips)

1/4 tsp cinnamon

salt to taste

*You can use ground beef or turkey if you prefer but you will get the optimal flavor and texture using the meat substitute. It makes superior chili, we swear!

**Açai juice can be found in the refrigerated section of health food grocers, or sold with the frozen foods as a pure fruit puree. If you can't find the ingredient, you can leave it out, but we think it is the key to this delicious stew.

1. Heat vegetable oil in a large stock pot.

2. Sauté onions and celery until soft, about 3 minutes.

3. Add garlic and sauté for an additional minute.

4. Add ground soy, chile powder, cumin and cayenne and sauté for 1 minute.

5. Stir in tomatoes, white beans vegetable broth, oregano, bay leaf and açai juice or fruit purée. Bring to a boil then simmer, covered, for 2 hours, stirring occasionally. If chili gets too thick, stir in water 1/2 cup at a time until chili reaches desired thickness.

6. Remove bay leaf and stir in chocolate and cinnamon. Turn off heat and season with salt to taste before serving.

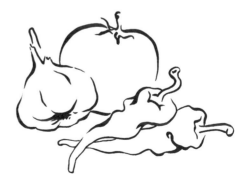

*Boost Your Libido*

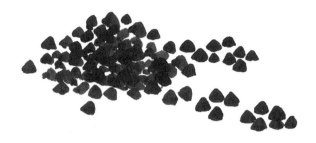

# handmade dark chocolate truffles

makes approximately 12 truffles

*Fact:* Studies show that a box of chocolates is considered a romantic gift.

*Love Diet truth:* Making the chocolates yourself almost guarantees you'll get lucky. Your lover won't guess it but dark chocolate truffles are one of the easiest candies you can possibly make. With these truffles we've swapped out the cream for half and half to cut some of the fat. And, by using premium dark chocolate, we've upped the dessert's antioxidant effects. Adding dried fruit to the center is our spin on a classic candy but it also helps to add libido-lifting impact to the treats. Just call them the gift that keeps on giving.

3 oz premium dark chocolate*

1/3 c half and half

2–3 tbsp your favorite dried fruit (blueberries, cherries, apricots and figs recommended)

cocoa powder for dusting

*You can use any dark chocolate bar or bitter-sweet baking chocolate to make this recipe, but we recommend using a chocolate that has at least 70% cocoa (it will tell the percentage on the label).

1. Grate chocolate or cut it into chip-sized pieces. (You can also use a premium chocolate chip.)

2. Heat half and half over medium high heat to a near boil. (Don't let it boil.)

3. Remove pan from heat and whisk in the chocolate, stirring until the mixture is completely smooth.

4. Cool in the refrigerator for about 3–4 hours (or overnight), until chocolate mixture has set.

5. Using a teaspoon, scoop cooled chocolate and form a ball, pressing 1 or 2 pieces of fruit into the center. (Don't waste your time trying to form your truffles into perfect spheres. A slightly uneven surface screams, "I rolled these chocolates with my own bare hands for your pleasure.") If the truffles wont hold shape, refrigerate chocolate mixture for another hour.

6. Cool the formed truffles in the refrigerator for about 5 minutes.

7. Roll each truffle in cocoa powder. Truffles will be soft but if they are so soft that the cocoa is absorbed, store in the refrigerator.

Truffles can be stored in a cool, dry place for up to 5 days.

*Boost Your Libido*

# basil-black pepper warming tea with cloves

vegetarian

*makes 1 serving*

Most of us buy our teas already packaged in neat little pouches. But its cheaper and almost as easy to make your own aphrodisiac herbal brew from ingredients in your spice cabinet and your garden. We invented this unusual combination with the goal of stirring up some body heat. This flavor trifecta also offers properties to sweeten breath, aid digestion and deliver a dose of antioxidants and vitamin A.

1. Crush the black peppercorns slightly so that they break into a few pieces (large enough that they won't slip through a strainer).

2. Put the peppercorns, cloves and chopped basil in a tea ball or strainer and steep in 5-6 oz hot water for 5 minutes or to desired strength.

For a sweet version, stir in a touch of honey or agave nectar before serving.

3 whole black peppercorns

3 whole cloves

3–4 fresh basil leaves, roughly chopped

# 4
# Quickies

You shouldn't give up on your diet just because you don't have the time (or desire) to cook. These are things we make in our homes for getting a healthy, libido-lifting meal on the table fast and with as little effort possible.

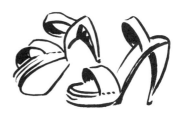

# fruit & yogurt
# pick-me-up parfait
vegetarian
*makes 1 parfait*

You really have no excuse to skip breakfast with a recipe this simple. And your libido is going to thank you for packing the most important meal of the day with super-ingredients like blueberries and yogurt.

1. Cut fruit of your choice (strawberries, raspberries, blackberries, peaches, pears, apricots, mangos or figs recommended), and toss with blueberries.

2. Put 1/2 cup fruit at the bottom of a parfait cup or small bowl.

3. Add 1/4 cup yogurt, spreading to cover fruit, and 1 tbsp granola or muesli.

4. Top with remaining fruit, then cover with yogurt. Sprinkle with remaining granola.

1/2 c your favorite fruit

1/2 c blueberries

1/2 c plain, Greek-style yogurt

2 tbsp your favorite granola or muesli

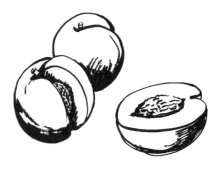

# rosemary tomato soup with a goat cheese crouton

vegetarian

*makes 4 servings*

You might think it's cheating to start from a box. We're not that big on processed foods but now that the soup companies have learned to get soup out of the can (with that piquant canniness that cannot be disguised), we're down with the occasional serving of soup-in-a-box. We just think it needs a little help from the herb garden. (If you have a favorite recipe and the time, by all means make your soup from scratch. It will be an especially fruitful endeavor when tomato season is at...well, its climax!)

4 c tomato soup

1 tbsp fresh rosemary, finely chopped

4 slices white or whole grain baguette, approx. 1/2" thick

olive oil for brushing

2–3 tbsp soft chèvre, (goat's milk cheese)

1. Add soup and rosemary to a pot and heat to a simmer.

2. Simmer for 5–10 minutes, stirring occasionally.

3. Lightly brush both sides of each slice of bread with olive oil.

4. While the soup is simmering, toast both sides of the bread in a sauté pan over medium heat, 2–3 minutes per side or until golden. (Bread can also be toasted in the oven.)

5. Spread one side of each slice of bread with a layer of chèvre.

6. Ladle hot soup into bowls and top each with a chèvre crouton.

# steamed artichokes with honey

*makes 2 servings*

Steamed artichokes are typically served with a creamy, calorie-laden dip. But you don't need all that fat. In fact, dips usually mask the artichoke's true flavor. So instead, we pair our artichokes with just a touch of honey, which simply augments their herbal flavors with an all-natural sweetness.

1. Fill a stock pot with approximately 1" of water. Cover the pot and bring the water to a boil, then turn the temperature down to low, keeping the pot covered.

2. Clean artichokes and cut the tops off so that if you turn them upside down, they will sit flat. Trim—but don't cut off—the stem. (Many people cut the stem off but this is one of the meatiest parts of the artichoke.) Then trim off any sharp, points on the ends of leaves.

3. Put the artichokes in the pot, stems facing up, so they sit flat, and steam for 20-30 minutes, until the leaves pull of easily. If the water runs low, add a small, additional amount.*

4. Transfer artichokes to a serving plate and serve with the honey for dipping.

2 artichokes
2–3 tbsp honey

*If you're in a rush, you can more quickly steam the artichokes in the microwave. Just be prepared for the outer leaves to discolor.

# crab salad with ripe avocado
*makes 2 servings*

Sometimes a simple salad fits the bill. The trick is to find the combination of ingredients that keeps the dish light but makes it satisfying. For us, crab salad with crunchy apples, salty bursts of capers and the creamy texture of avocados does the job. The crab mixture also works well as a dip. Just mash the avocado and blend it in to give the dip a smooth texture and serve with pita chips, page 113 or raw veggies and fruits.

5 oz crab meat or a 6 oz can of crab, drained

1/2 crisp, red apple, (such as a Fuji or Braeburn), cored, (skin on), and finely chopped

1 tbsp celery, finely chopped

1 tbsp sweet onion, (such as Vidalia), finely chopped

1 1/2 tsp capers, drained

1 1/2 tbsp cream cheese, softened

1 tsp Dijon mustard

1/4 tsp salt

1 tsp fresh chives, minced

2 c baby greens

1/2 avocado, thinly sliced

wedge of fresh lemon

1. In a small mixing bowl, combine crab, apple, celery, onion, capers, cream cheese and Dijon, mixing thoroughly.

2. Season with salt then gently fold in chives.

3. Evenly divide the greens between 2 plates. Top with the crab and garnish plates with the avocado. Squeeze fresh lemon juice over both salads before serving.

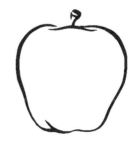

*Quickies*

# vegetarian albondigas (spanish meatballs)

vegetarian

*makes 4 servings*

Meatballs are a popular part of Spanish tapas. Our version uses another popular Spanish tradition: wine. Because we layer the meatballs with additional flavors, we think its fine to use ready-made. To make this super-quick appetizer even healthier, we buy veggie meatballs (which tend to have more flavor and don't leave the onions coated in fat like pork and beef will). You can, of course, use any kind of meatball you like but, just for us, try the veggie at least once.

1. Over medium heat, coat the bottom of a small stock pan with oil. Sautéé the onion until soft, about 2 minutes.

2. Add the meatballs to the pot and sauté until brown on at least 2 sides (an additional 2 or 3 minutes).

3. Add white wine and turn temperature to low. Simmer, covered, for 15 minutes.

4. Remove from heat and transfer meatballs and onions to a serving dish with a slotted spoon. (Meatballs will be very moist. Move them gently to ensure you don't wind up with a pile of ground soy.)

2 tsp olive oil

1 spanish onion, roughly chopped

16 frozen vegetarian meatballs*

1 c dry white wine

1 tbsp flat leaf parsley, finely chopped

* The recipe also works with turkey, pork and beef meatballs but we love the clean flavor and health benefits of the soy variety.

5. Sprinkle parsley over meatballs as a garnish.

Remaining liquid can be discarded or used as a sauce for simple baked or seared fish.

Since Albondigas is a Spanish tradition, try simmering the meatballs in a dry, Spanish white wine, like an Albariño, then enjoy the rest of the bottle as your effort's reward.

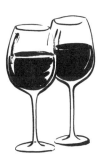

# tomato-anchovy bruschetta with a side of "naked" pasta

*makes 4 servings*

In a previous life as a waiter, I made tableside Caesar salads and folks would say "Oh! no anchovies," then would proceed to tell me that the Caesar "didn't taste right." Duh! Anchovies are what give a Caesar its signature tangy/salty goodness. And guess what? They're GREAT for you. In my house, anchovy toast is one of those dishes everyone fights over. I typically serve it on toasted baguette slices with a bowl of "naked" pasta. But the anchovy mixture will also rock your favorite pasta as a substitute for a traditional sauce. I've noted a bunch of optional ingredients that I think work well with the dish so you can pick, choose and find your own style.

—Juan-Carlos

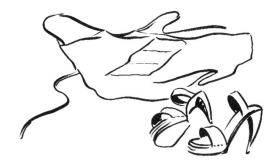

2 tins anchovies in oil

1 tsp olive oil

1 lg shallot, minced

2 large, ripe tomatoes, diced

1 tbsp lemon juice

pepper to taste

8 oz whole wheat or brown rice pasta

1 tbsp high-quality olive oil

2–3 tbsp Parmesan or your favorite grating cheese

1/2 c ripe tomatoes, chopped for the pasta, (optional)

2 tbsp minced basil, (optional)

1/2 baguette, sliced in 1/8"-thick rounds then toasted

*Feel free to add any and all of your favorite steamed or sautéed vegetables to the pasta dish, including broccoli, broccoli rabe, peppers, fennel, artichokes, etc.

1. Drain and discard the oil from the anchovy tins, then finely chop anchovies.

2. Heat the olive oil in a small, nonstick sauté pan over medium heat.

3. Add the shallot and sauté until translucent, about 1–2 minutes.

4. Add the anchovies to the pan and heat through.

5. Stir in half the diced tomatoes and cook until tomatoes are just soft, 2–3 minutes.

6. Remove pan from heat and toss in the other half of the diced tomatoes.

7. Bring water for pasta to a boil and cook according to package instructions.

8. Toss cooked pasta with olive oil and (optional) tomatoes and basil then top with cheese.*

9. Serve anchovy mixture spread on baguette slices with the pasta on the side. (You can also top pasta with the anchovies and serve the toast, brushed with a little olive oil, on the side.)

# stove top sous vide salmon with fennel-apricot slaw
makes 4 servings

Sous vide, French for "under vacuum," is a cooking method gaining popularity in the "molecular gastronomy," fine dining craze. While true sous vide cooking requires an expensive piece of equipment called a thermal circulator, there is a way to take the core idea of sous vide cooking (slowly poaching a protein—in this case fish—in a vacuum sealed bag to lock in moisture and flavor) and use the concept at home in a low-tech guise. (You will not quite get the same effect as you would from a thermal circulator because this piece of equipment actually stirs the water, guaranteeing even cooking. But we think, with salmon, anyway, the results of our method are sufficiently satisfying and make a fine introduction to this low-fat, high snob appeal style of cooking.)

We use a small vacuum sealer for this recipe—if you are looking for a gadget worth an investment, this is definitely one to consider; a vacuum sealer has a multitude of uses. But you can get almost the same effect from tight plastic wrap sealing.

It may seem strange that we've chosen a dish using slow poaching as a "quickie" but we think the finished dish's complexity of flavor and level of presentation offer pretty fabulous return on investment for the amount of prep time. And since your hands are free while the fish poaches, the possibility of a *pre*dinner quickie isn't out of the question!

12 oz wild salmon, 1/2"–3/4" thickness

salt and pepper to taste

1 garlic clove, peeled and sliced

1 small lemon, sliced into rounds

1 fennel bulb

1/2 c Vidalia or other sweet onion

6 dried apricots

1 tbsp lemon zest

2 tsp grape seed or other neutral oil

2 tbsp apple cider vinegar

4 tsp salmon roe, (or more if desired)

1. Place a pot of water over a burner and heat to 113 degrees, checking constantly with a thermometer.

2. Season salmon with salt and pepper and place in a vacuum sealer bag with the garlic and lemon. Vacuum seal the bag shut. (If you do not own a vacuum sealer, tightly wrap salmon, garlic and lemon in a layer of plastic wrap. Prick the plastic wrap and press out any air. Cut a second piece of plastic wrap that is at least twice the length of the fish. Wrap the parcel in the second piece of plastic wrap so that the ends will fold over the opposite sides of the first piece of plastic wrap. (This is to help ensure the package stays watertight. Pull wrap as tightly as you can before sealing ends.)

3. Submerge fish parcel in the 113 degree water.

4. Get a cup of ice and keep it by within reach while you monitor the water temperature. If temperature gets above 123 degrees, drop ice into water, one cube at a time until temperature returns to 113 degrees (but not below). Cook, monitoring in this fashion for 15-20 minutes, depending on thickness of salmon fillets. (The thicker the steak, the longer it should cook. If you like your fish on the rare side, cook for less minutes. If you prefer your fish cooked through, cook for the full poaching time.)

5. Take packet from water and remove fish, discarding garlic and lemon.

*for the fennel-apricot slaw:*

1. Using a food processor or mandolin, shave fennel and onion into paper-thin slices, reserving the dill-like fennel tops (fronds).

2. Finely chop apricots and mix in a bowl with fennel and onions. Add zest, oil and vinegar and toss until fennel is thoroughly coated.

3. Add in 1 tbsp of fennel fronds for color and season with salt and pepper to taste. (Fennel and onions can be prepped a day in advance, but step 3 should be reserved until serving.)

*to serve:*

Place 1/4 of the slaw on each of 2 plates (sprinkle with fronds and season with salt and pepper if this was not done in advance). Top with 3 oz salmon and garnish each with 1 tsp salmon roe.

Salmon with Pinot Noir is a much-loved pairing among the food and wine "elite." We recommend trying the combination, especially since Pinot Noir has some of the highest levels of resveratrol of all wines. (Resveratrol is the famously heart-healthy compound found in red wines.)

Store remaining fish, roe and slaw in separate containers and plate at the last minute. Leftover fish can be served cold, or gently rewarmed before serving.

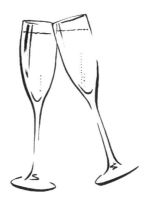

# rosewater-scented champagne
*makes 2 drinks*

This is one of our simplest tricks for delivering a complex cocktail. Sparkling wine is already layered with interesting attributes from its icy chill to its effervescence and bright array of flavors. By adding just a trace of rosewater, you're emphasizing the Champagne's aphrodisiac attributes while allowing the wine's natural flavors to still shine.

2–4 drops rosewater

10 oz Champagne or sparkling wine

1. Place 1–2 drops rosewater into each of 2 Champagne flutes. (For added ease, use an eye dropper.)

2. Top each with 5 oz Champagne or sparkling wine.

3. Drink.

*Quickies*

# cmp fondue

*serves 2*

My great grandmother Amy (for whom I was named), owned an ice cream parlor. One of her most popular items was the CMP sundae (chocolate, marshmallow and peanuts). I think this ice cream dish is a mid Atlantic specialty, because I've never seen a CMP outside of Pennsylvania. In this recipe, we've eliminated the ice cream and have gone straight for the good stuff. (We've also layered the chocolate flavor with a healthy dose of cacao nibs—nibs are the chocolate at its most pure and are loaded with antioxidants as well as a terrific, crunchy texture.) By turning the CMP into a fondue, it becomes an interactive dish, one that is fun for sharing, feeding and foreplay.—Amy

2 tbsp roasted, salted peanuts, finely chopped*

1 tbsp butter

1/4 c dark chocolate chips

1 tsp light corn syrup

1/2 tsp vanilla

2 tsp cacao nibs**

8 marshmallows

1. Put peanuts in a shallow bowl.

2. In a double boiler over hot (not boiling) water, melt butter. Stir in chocolate and corn syrup, stirring constantly until melted.

3. Remove from heat and add vanilla and nibs.

4. Dip marshmallows first in the chocolate, then roll in the peanuts. Eat immediately to enjoy the melty, crunchy combo.

If you aren't planning to serve immediately, transfer chocolate to a fondue pot to keep warm.

*Variation:* Place 1/2 fresh strawberry and 1 mini marshmallow on a toothpick or skewer. Dip in chocolate and peanuts for a juicy, summery variation on the dessert.

*If you are trying to watch your sodium intake, use unsalted peanuts and sprinkle them with a pinch of coarse sea salt.

**Cocoa nibs are sold in gourmet cooking stores like Sur La Table, gourmet grocers and online.

# 5
# Romantic
# Weekends

Most of this book is about *you* and your health. This chapter is about sharing. We don't expect you to make these foods every day. Some of our Romantic Weekend recipes require complex preparations, others use expensive or higher-calorie ingredients. But they're those fun things you pack on a picnic, make for a dinner party, birthday, anniversary or just because you need it. Of all of our recipes, we think of these as the social foods—things you want to eat yourself but taste better when they're shared.

# whole grain french toast with warm blueberry sauce

vegetarian

*makes 2 servings*

I love french toast, always have—as breakfast, lunch or dinner. By making your French toast with whole grain bread, you add texture and up the nutritional content. Those who know me as Pastry Chef Juan-Carlos are not going to be surprised that I like my French toast sweet. So the agave nectar in the batter is the bump to satisfy my sweet tooth. You can experiment with different sweeteners or omit it if you like.—Juan-Carlos

1. Whisk together the egg whites, egg beaters, cinnamon and agave in a shallow bowl. Set aside.

2. Heat a large, nonstick sauté pan over medium heat. Lightly spray the pan with a nonstick cooking spray (butter-flavored recommended).

3. Dip both sides of the bread into the egg mixture 1 slice at a time. Do not soak the bread or allow it to get soggy.

4. Place the slices into the heated sauté pan and cook until golden on the first side, about 1 1/2 minutes, then flip and cook 1 additional minute or until golden.

5. Serve with blueberry sauce (page 69) or, if you prefer, your favorite syrup.

2 egg whites

1/4 c egg beaters or other liquid eggs

1/4 tsp cinnamon

1/2 tsp agave nectar*

4 slices whole grain or whole wheat bread

blueberry sauce, (page 69)

*Agave nectar is a natural, liquid sweetener that can be found at health food stores. If you don't have agave nectar, you can use honey, although it will slightly alter the taste.

*for the blueberry sauce:*

1 c frozen blueberries

1/2 c orange juice

2 tbsp sugar

fresh blueberries to garnish, (optional)

*for the blueberry sauce:*

1. Combine all ingredients in a small saucepan over medium heat and bring to a simmer. Turn the temperature to low and simmer until all blueberries have popped and the sauce has a syrupy consistency, about 15 minutes.

2. If the sauce is too tart, add a little extra sugar to the simmering syrup, stirring until completely dissolved.

Use leftover sauce to top pancakes, ice cream, pound cake or mix into plain yogurt.

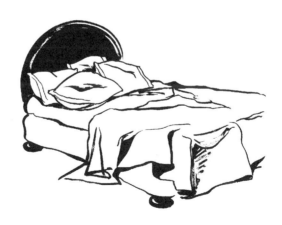

# garden tomato & avocado picnic sandwiches

vegetarian
makes 2 sandwiches

I was first introduced to the tomato-avocado sandwich combo in Australia. I liked the flavors so much that I made an art of perfecting this picnic food. I think the sandwich tastes best using a perfectly ripe, Brandywine heirloom tomato, Haas avocado and super-crunchy, seed bread. But it works with any tomato, avocado and whole grain, so long as the tomato is in season and ripe. You're going to be tempted to omit the butter. Don't do it. The thin layer of butter acts as a barrier between tomato and bread, preventing your masterpiece from going all soggy.—Amy

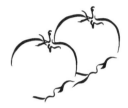

1. Thinly spread 2 slices of bread with the butter. (Use just enough butter to cover the slice.)

2. Top each buttered slice with tomato slices.

3. Sprinkle the tomato with salt and pepper to taste.

4. Remove skin from the avocado and mash to a chunky paste.

5. Spread half the avocacdo on each of the 2 remaining bread slices.

6. Form sandwiches, cut in half and either serve immediately or pack up for a picnic. (Sandwiches will last for about 4 hours.)

4 slices whole grain bread

1–1 1/2 tsp whipped or softened butter

10 thin slices garden tomato, (about 1 medium tomato)

1/2 avocado

salt and black pepper to taste

# lobster pasta in champagne tarragon sauce

*makes 2 servings*

4 oz dried buckwheat (soba) or whole wheat noodles

2 tsp unsalted butter

1 shallot, minced

2/3 c sparkling wine

1 tbsp fresh tarragon or 3/4 tsp dried

1 tbsp fresh lemon juice

5–6 oz lobster, (approximately 1 large tail), cut into bite-sized pieces

1 c fresh arugula

2 tbsp crème fraîche

salt to taste

2 tsp flying fish caviar (tobiko)*

*Tobiko is sold in Asian food stores, specialty grocery and most grocery stores with a sushi department. If you can't find it at any of these stores, try buying it from a sushi restaurant.

If there's anything that could improve upon lobster, it would have to be Champagne and tarragon butter. This is one of our most decadent recipes, so don't go halfway. Invest in the highest-quality ingredients, cook with love and serve aside chilled flutes of something bubbly. (You might also want to clear your calendar. If your lover likes lobster, you're going to be busy for awhile.)

1. Bring a pot of water to a boil. Cook pasta according to package instructions.

2. Melt butter in a nonstick sauté pan over medium heat. Sauté shallot until soft, about 1–2 minutes. Add sparkling wine, tarragon and lemon juice and bring to a simmer.

3. Turn heat to medium-low and add lobster, simmering until cooked through, about 5 minutes.

4. Remove from heat and immediately add arugula, tossing until it begins to wilt.

5. Season with salt to taste.

*to serve:*

Divide pasta between 2 plates. Top each with half of the lobster and sauce. Garnish with 1 tbsp crème fraîche with 1 tsp of flying fish roe.

# seared halibut with mushroom "cream" on a bed of braised celery

makes 4 servings

Most people think its crazy to use soymilk in place of cream. But soymilk has a sweetness and silky quality not dissimilar to cream. And since this recipe uses so little, you can serve it at a dinner party and we doubt any of your guests will ever notice that what they're tasting is soy. Like soy, celery has plant estrogens, making this dish a great choice for the ladies.

1. Wash, trim and slice mushrooms.

2. Heat butter in a sauté pan over medium heat.

3. Sauté shallots for 1 minute.

4. Add mushrooms and a pinch of salt to the pan and sauté for 3 minutes.

5. Turn the heat to low, add the soymilk and simmer for 4 minutes, stirring occasionally.

6. Sprinkle both sides of the halibut with salt and pepper.

7. Sear the halibut over medium heat in a nonstick pan coated with cooking spray. Cook for 3–4 minutes per side, turning once.

8. To serve, put 4 celery pieces on each plate. Top with a halibut steak and 1/4 of the mushroom mix-

1 lb button or crimini mushrooms*

1 tsp unsalted butter

1 shallot, finely chopped

1 pinch salt

1/4 c soymilk

4 halibut steaks, 4 oz each

salt and pepper

1 batch braised celery, (below)

1 tbsp parsley, finely chopped

*For a more exotic taste, use 1/2 lb button or crimini and 1/2 lb shitake, chanterelle or morel mushrooms.

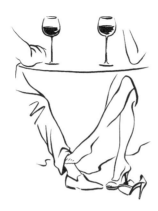

ture, making sure to spoon a little cream over each steak. Garnish with parsley.

We also like to serve mushroom "cream" over baked chicken breasts, seared salmon and roasted loin of pork.

*for the braised celery:*
8 stalks celery
2 tsp unsalted butter
1/2 c vegetable stock

*for the braised celery:*

1. Trim celery and cut each stalk in half on a diagonal.

2. Melt butter in a sauté pan over medium heat. Sauté celery for 3 minutes.

3. Add in stock and simmer, covered, for 5 minutes.

4. Uncover and cook for an additional 3 minutes.

Braised celery is also a great accompaniment to simple, grilled seafoods and wild game.

# tea smoked pork & shitakes with a rhubarb purée

*makes 4 servings*

Smoking on the stovetop is one of my favorite—not to mention most healthy—cooking techniques. I use it with all kinds of fish and meat. Once you get the hang of the method, try it with another meat and maybe throw in some tomatoes. (While you're at it, try a different tea.) The best part about stovetop smoking is the cleanup. Before you start, thoroughly wrap your pan in foil then, once everything has cooled, just pull it from the pan straight to the trash.—Juan-Carlos

*You will need 3 things for this recipe. A pan, or wok, with a lid, a rack that fits inside the pan, and a whole lot of aluminum foil. If you don't have a rack the right size, try using a wok screen or even the rack of a toaster oven.*

1. Line pan with aluminum foil.

2. Mix rice, sugar and tea together then sprinkle the mixture on the bottom of the pan.

3. Place pan on a burner over high heat.

4. When sugar begins to melt and smoke, turn the heat to medium.

5. Suspend rack over the sugar. (If the rack does not fit conveniently, you can make 4 balls of crumpled aluminum foil placed right on top of the sugar as a prop for the rack.)

1/2 c plain rice

1 c brown sugar

1/4 c loose leaf apricot or peach black tea blend

1 lb pork loin, (or 4 loin chops weighing about 1 lb)

salt and pepper

8 shitake mushrooms, ends trimmed

1 batch rhubarb purée, (page 75)

6. If you are using a pork loin, cut into 4 evenly-sized servings. Season both sides of the meat with salt and pepper and place on rack along with the shitake mushrooms. Cover tightly with the lid.

7. Allow pork to smoke for approximately 15–20 minutes, depending on thickness. (Cuts of a 1 inch or greater thickness will take up to 20 minutes, less for thinner cuts.) Chops should seem firm but not dry. To double check, make a slice in the center of one chop. If there is any pink, continue to cook.

8. Serve over the rhubarb puree, or dress with your favorite vinaigrette and serve with steamed greens.

*for the rhubarb purée:*

1 shallot

2 tbsp water

1 tbsp and 1 tsp balsamic vinegar

3 tbsp sugar

2 c fresh rhubarb, about 3 stalks, leaves discarded, ends trimmed

*for the rhubarb purée:*

1. In a nonstick saucepan over medium heat, sauté shallot for 1 minute.

2. Add water and balsamic vinegar to the pot and scrape any stuck bits of shallot from the bottom.

3. Stir in sugar and rhubarb.

4. Bring to a simmer and reduce heat to low.

5. Simmer, uncovered, until rhubarb is fork tender, about 14–15 minutes.

6. Remove from heat and stir until rhubarb breaks apart and makes a thick purée.

7. Allow purée to cool for 1 hour to set.

Store in the refrigerator and warm to room temperature to serve.

*Romantic Weekends*

# cupid's kiss champagne cocktail

*makes 2 servings*

I originally created this drink for a hotel's Valentine's promotion. We wanted something that was red, could be prepped in advance and was low enough in alcohol that guests could enjoy a couple and still manage a... ahem, command performance when they returned to their rooms. If Champagne isn't your thing, the fruit syrup works well as an addition to a vodka and soda. And unlike most sweetened, alcoholic drinks, it incorporates some good-for-you ingredients without a calorie overload.—Amy

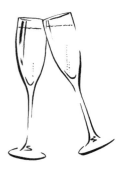

1. Add 1 tbsp fruit syrup to a Champagne flute, top with the Champagne or sparkling wine.

2. Drain and repeat.

2 tbsp balsamic fruit syrup

10 oz Brut Champagne or sparkling wine

*for the balsamic fruit syrup*

1. Marinate fruit and 3 tbsp sugar in the balsamic for 30 minutes–1 hour.

2. Taste mixture, and if it is not sweet enough, stir in additional sugar 1 tsp at a time, up to 3 tsp, allowing fruit to marinate for an additional 10 minutes.

3. Strain to remove seeds, pressing fruit against the strainer to release all the juice. Store juice in the refrigerator until serving. (The macerated fruit remaining in the strainer can be saved in a separate container to serve over ice cream or use as the topping on Bedtime Yogurt, page 120.)

*for the balsamic fruit syrup:*

1/2 c thawed frozen raspberries

1/2 c thawed frozen strawberries

3-4 tbsp granulated sugar

2 tbsp balsamic vinegar

# hot chocolate martini

*makes 2 servings*

We decided to see what would happen if we took the sophistication of a martini, the comfort of a childhood favorite like hot chocolate and swirled it all together. We're pretty sweet on the results and with the addition of the cocoa rim, the presentation is a big hit with our friends.

cocoa powder for the rim

1 c hot soymilk, (or regular milk)

1 tbsp dark chocolate, grated

1 oz vanilla vodka

2 oz chocolate vodka

1. Put a small amount of cocoa powder on a plate or saucer. Wet the rim of two martini glasses with soymilk. Roll the rim in the cocoa to make an even coating around the whole rim.

2. Add dark chocolate to the hot soymilk, stirring until melted. (You can use any candy counter chocolate but we recommend choosing a bar with a high percentage of cocoa, 65% or 70% is good, for a really rich, chocolate flavor.)

3. Stir in vanilla and chocolate vodkas then pour into 2 martini glasses. Serve immediately.

*Romantic Weekends*

# individual rosemary & citrus custard cakes

vegetarian

*makes 4 cakes*

What's impressive about these tart, little desserts is that they magically separate into cake and custard layers in the oven—all on their own! Despite being relatively low-calorie, their flavors are complex. You might never have thought of adding rosemary to a dessert but used in a small amount, it adds an interesting herbal—but not savory—dimension.

1. Preheat oven to 350 degrees.

2. Coat 4 individual custard or soufflé cups with non-stick cooking spray.

3. Separate eggs. Make sure the egg whites are at, or close to, room temperature or you'll never achieve the desired fluffy clouds you are about to create.

4. Beat the whites to a foamy state, then slowly add in 1/2 cup sugar while continuing to beat until glossy, soft peaks form. (Do not over beat.)

5. In a separate bowl, combine remaining sugar with butter and beat until thoroughly mixed.

6. Add flour, citrus juice, zest, rosemary and salt to the butter and sugar mixture. Beat at a medium-high speed until thoroughly blended.

7. Stir in egg yolks and milk to form a batter.

2 large eggs, room temperature

1/4 c and 2 tsp granulated sugar

1 tbsp butter, softened

3 tbsp all-purpose flour

3 tbsp lemon juice

2 tsp tangerine juice

1/2 tsp lemon zest

1/4 tsp tangerine zest

1 tsp rosemary, minced

1/4 tsp salt

3/4 c and 2 tsp 1% or 2% milk*

*You can use skim milk for the recipe but we find that the small amount of fat improves the texture of both the custard and cake portions of the dish.

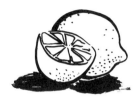

8. Fold 1/4 of the soft peaked egg whites into the batter. With gentle strokes, continue to gradually fold in the egg whites until all the whites have been combine into the batter. If you handle the egg whites roughly, you will lose the ethereal quality of the final cakes.

9. Divide the batter among the 4 cups.

10. Place the cups in a shallow baking dish with about an inch 1" warm water. The water will allow the cakes to steam and rise gently in the oven.

11. Bake the cakes for 35 minutes or until the custards are set and the tops lightly golden.

12. Remove cups from pan. Chill for at least 30 minutes or until cups feel cold and custard is completely set.

13. To serve, invert the cakes onto individual plates. The bottom of each cake will be a light angel food topped by a golden custard dome.

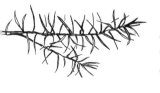

Because they aren't very sweet, we like serving these cakes with a dry white wine like a Sauvignon Blanc or a Chardonnay. It really adds to the unexpected element of the whole dessert.

# decadent chocolate layer cake with cream cheese frosting

### vegetarian
*makes 10–12 servings*

This rich, moist, multilayered cake is Amy's favorite (and far lower in calories than you'd ever guess). It is actually a variation on a vegan cake recipe created by Chrysta Wilson for her Kiss My Bundt Bakery. But instead of topping the cake with vegan buttercream, we arrange it in 4 layers, sandwiched with light cream cheese frosting. The result is not only visually impressive, the super-moist cake—made even more moist by the layers of cream cheese—is as rich as fudge and, we think, as satisfying. Unlike most baked goods, this one gets better with age. Store in the refrigerator and serve 24 hours after frosting for a total cakegasm.

1 3/4 c sugar*

2 c all-purpose flour

3/4 c high-fat cocoa powder**

1 1/4 tsp baking powder

1 1/4 tsp baking soda

3/4 tsp salt

1 c unsweetened soymilk

1/3 c vegetable oil

2 tsp vanilla extract

2 tbsp instant coffee granules

3/4 c water, boiling

1. Preheat oven to 350 degrees.

2. Sift together sugar, flour, cocoa powder, baking powder, baking soda and salt. Set aside.

3. Add soymilk, oil and vanilla to a mixing bowl. Using an electric mixer, beat on medium speed for 1 minute.

4. With the mixer on low speed, add dry ingredients to the wet, 1/2 cup at a time. Do this slowly so that the batter doesn't become lumpy.

5. When thoroughly combined, dissolve instant coffee granules into the boiling water. Slowly mix the boiling coffee into the batter by hand, stirring until completely combined. Note: the batter will be thin.

*To make a vegan version of the cake, simply use vegan sugar, found at most health food stores. To make a vegan frosting, use vegan powdered sugar and a nondairy cream cheese substitute.

**We recommend using a high-fat cocoa powder for an intense chocolate flavor. We like Callebaut among the high-end brands and on the less expensive end, there's Hershey's Special Dark.

6. Transfer batter to cake 2 round cake pans that have been coated with a baker's cooking spray that includes flour (or greased and floured).

7. Bake cakes until an inserted toothpick or cake tester comes out clean—about 18–23 minutes (time may vary by oven).

8. Invert cakes onto a cooling rack or serving plate. If cakes resists, cool in the pan for 15 minutes before inverting. Cool completely before frosting.

*for the frosting:*

3 oz unsalted butter, softened

8 oz Neufchatel cream cheese, softened

2 C powdered sugar, sifted

1/2 tsp vanilla extract

*for the frosting:*

1. With an electric mixer on a medium speed, cream the butter and the cream cheese until soft and completely smooth, about 2–3 minutes.

2. Turn the mixer speed to low and slowly add the powdered sugar 1/2 cup at a time, making sure to scrape down any frosting stuck to the sides of the bowl.

3. When sugar is fully incorporated, add vanilla extract.

4. Mix on a medium speed until frosting is smooth and fluffy.

*to assemble:*

1. Slice each of the cakes into 2 rounds (so that you will have 4 layers in total). You can cut the cakes with a bread knife, but to easily cut the cakes into nearly perfect disks, stick a toothpick horizontally

into the side of the cake half-way from the top of the round. Take a 20" piece of unflavored, wax-free dental floss. Wrap the floss around the cake just above your toothpick marker. Cross the floss as if you were tying a bow. Keep pulling the floss until the floss has cut the entire first layer.

2. Repeat with the second round.

3. Spread 1/4 of the frosting evenly across the top of the first round (the one on your serving plate). Do NOT ice down the sides of the cake or you will run out of frosting.

4. Top with a cake round and frost the top of this round, repeating with the third round.

5. Add the top layer of cake and spread a very thin layer of frosting. This is your "crumb coat." (The crumb coat will help prevent specks of dark cake in the white frosting on the finished cake.) Refrigerate cake for 15–30 minutes then frost the top of the cake with the remaining frosting.

# 7
# Little Blue Pill Foods

Some foods are declared aphrodisiac because of an immediate, physiological effect. (Chiles and ginger raise body temperature and promote adrenalin, coffee elevates mood and offers instant energy, etc.) This chapter features those kinds of foods, incorporated into recipes suitable for that night you intend to seal the deal, the weekend the kids go to grandma's or when your flame needs reigniting. *(Four out of five recipe testers using this chapter report utter satisfaction!)*

# love me tender
# peanut butter omelet

vegetarian

*makes 2 servings*

Elvis brought us the pb/banana combo and he was one smoldering dude so surely the pairing can help the rest of us. A peanut butter omelet may sound crazy but we know it works because we stole the idea from a breakfast joint on Cape Cod. The egg acts almost like bread but offers protein for energy. The chili in the peanut butter sauce really heats things up, and the bananas? Ever wonder where the phrase "going bananas" originated? Mmm hmm, time to take another look at the yellow love fruit.

1. In a small mixing bowl, whisk eggs and egg whites until mixture is thoroughly combined and slightly foamy. Stir in salt.

2. Either divide the beaten eggs into 2 servings to cook 1 at a time or make 1 omelet to share, (we vote for the share technique!).

3. In a small pan, melt the butter and swirl pan to coat the entire bottom. (If you are going to make 2 omelets, divide the butter between 2 pans.)

4. Cook the eggs as you would any omelet, drizzling the peanut butter sauce over both servings when the eggs begin to set.

2 eggs*

3 egg whites*

pinch salt

2 tsp butter

1 banana, sliced into rounds

1/2 tsp fresh parsley, finely chopped

2-3 tbsp peanut butter sauce, (recipe below)

*You can substitute Egg Beaters for the eggs and egg whites.

5. When the omelet is almost cooked, top half the pan with the chopped banana and parsley then fold the other half over top.

6. Slide the omelet to your serving pan and enjoy. Make it a full meal by adding a couple pieces of smoky turkey bacon and slices of your favorite fresh fruit.

*for the peanut sauce:*

3 tbsp smooth peanut butter, room temperature, (or soften in microwave if it has been refrigerated)

3/4 tsp soy sauce

1 tsp rice wine vinegar

1/4 tsp sriracha (hot chili sauce)

2-3 tbsp hot water

*for the peanut sauce:*

1. Whisk the peanut butter, soy sauce, rice wine vinegar and sriracha together in a mixing bowl.

2. Slowly add hot water to thin mixture. You may not need to use all of the water.

Leftover peanut sauce makes a tongue tingling, libido lifting dip for chicken, tofu skewers or fresh spring rolls.

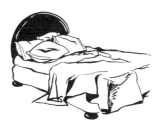

*Little Blue Pill Foods*

# morning after date shake
vegetarian

*makes 2 servings*

We've heard that the recommendation for milk-soaked dates served as an aphrodisiac originated with the Kama Sutra. We're not sure why. But what we do know is that dates are a source of magnesium—essential for sexual hormone production—and are a great source of fiber. Best of all, if bloggers are to be believed, there are few hangover cures that beat a good date shake. So live it up; just be sure to prep the dates at night for a long, slow morning in bed.

1. Pit and chop dates and soak overnight in the milk.

2. Combine graham cracker crumbs and 1 pinch cardamom in a shallow dish or plate. Moisten the top of 2 glasses with milk then dip rims of both glasses in the crumb mixture.

3. Put dates and soaking milk in blender. Add yogurt, honey, 1 pinch cardamom, ice and blend.

4. Carefully pour liquid into the 2 rimmed glasses. Tastes best drunk in bed.

5 dried dates, soaked in milk, (prepped in advance)

1 graham cracker, crushed into crumbs or 1 tbsp graham cracker crumbs

2 pinches cardamom*

1/2 c plain, Greek-style yogurt

1 tsp honey

8 ice cubes

*A tiny amount of cardamom can really dominate this shake. Be careful not to over-season by measuring a pinch as a scant 1/8 tsp.

# red curry shrimp with ripe mango

*makes 2–3 servings*

Hailing from the Caribbean (I was born in the Dominican Republic), I grew up on seafood and tropical fruit. Many people are surprised to see a Caribbean dish with Indian flavors. But more than a few from the subcontinent came to the islands seeking their fortune, bringing their tastes with them. This recipe is a great choice for anyone sensitive to spicy flavors, as it is warming without an aggressive bite. The addition of cold, sweet mango at the end seals the deal. —Juan-Carlos

1/2 ripe mango

12 large shrimp

pinch salt

1 tsp paprika

1/2 tsp coriander powder

1/4 tsp cumin

1/4 tsp black pepper, freshly ground

1/4 tsp cinnamon

1/2 tsp powdered ginger

1 tbsp grape seed or other neutral oil

1 small red onion, diced

1 large tomato, diced

1. Peel and dice mango then chill in the refrigerator

2. Peel the shrimp and sprinkle with a pinch of salt.

3. In a small mixing bowl, combine paprika, coriander, cumin, black pepper, cinnamon and ginger. Add shrimp and toss until well coated.

4. Heat oil in a nonstick sauté pan over high heat.

5. Add shrimp to pan and sauté until they begin to curl and change color.

6. Add the onion and tomato and continue to cook for an additional 2 minutes, tossing occasionally. (Onions should still have some crunch.)

7. Remove from heat and transfer to a serving platter. Top with cold mango and serve immediately for a hot/cold/spicy/sweet sensation.

Leftovers are delicious over Bibb or Romaine as a cold salad.

*Little Blue Pill Foods*

# coffee-kissed buffalo burgers

*makes 4 burgers*

Buffalo makes a great alternative to beef. It's lower than beef in cholesterol and calories, higher in protein and iron. You may not consciously realize it but these are things your libido wants. Most buffalo is raised grazing on grass instead of manufactured feed and synthetic hormones. Which means it also *isn't* delivering crud your body *doesn't* want. (Ever took a minute to think about what beef cattle eat on a feedlot? We'll tell you one thing, it's not fresh grass.)

1. Mix salt, pepper and coffee grounds into the ground buffalo and form 4 burger patties with 1/4 inch thickness.

2. Brush grill with cooking oil and heat to high.

3. Cook burgers for 3–5 minutes per side depending on desired doneness, flipping once. (Because of its low fat content, buffalo will become tough if overcooked.)

4. After burgers are flipped, add onion rounds to the grill. Grill onions on 2–3 minutes per side.

5. Top each half of the buns with 1–2 tsp oyster sauce. Add a tomato slice (optional) and 1/4 of the grilled onions. Top with a burger and serve openfaced.

1/2 tsp salt

1/2 tsp pepper

2 tsp fine coffee grounds

1 lb ground buffalo, (or 4 buffalo patties)

1/2 sweet onion, cut into rounds

2 tbsp oyster sauce

4 slices ripe tomato, (optional)

2 whole grain sandwich rolls

If you are only serving 2 burgers, save the second bun and toppings separately, in the refrigerator, for up to 48 hours.

The ground buffalo mixture can also be used to make meatballs. Just brown lightly in a sauté pan and serve with pasta or as an appetizer with oyster sauce for dipping.

It is well known that a big, bold red wine can take a burger to new aphrodisiac heights. But because we love the unexpected, we recommend trying your burger with a glass of something light and fresh like a Riesling. We think the effect of a bright, white wine dancing across the tongue and washing down the heavier meat has the ability to awaken the senses in a deliciously surprising manner.

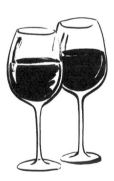

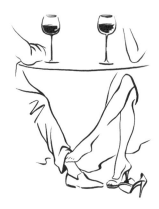

# hot sausage stew
makes 4 servings

We don't really have to tell you why hot sausage gets the libido going, do we? Well, rather than stating the obvious, we'd like to mention that fennel, one of the stew's main flavorings, is a source of magnesium, iron, vitamin C and manganese.

1. Brush grill with olive oil and heat to medium. Grill sausages, turning occasionally until all sides are done, about 12 minutes in total. (Cooking times may vary depending on the sausages.) Remove from heat and set aside.

2.  Spray a large, nonstick pan with cooking spray and heat to medium-high. Sauté onion until soft, about 3 minutes.

olive oil for brushing grill

4 Italian-style chicken or turkey sausages

1 red onion, thinly sliced into rounds

1 red bell pepper, cored and thinly sliced

1 yellow bell pepper, cored and thinly sliced

1 small fennel bulb, trimmed and thinly sliced (like the onion)

1 tsp paprika

1/2 tsp ground coriander

1/4 tsp salt

1/4 tsp black pepper

2 cloves garlic, finely minced

1 1/2 c dry red wine*

2 tbsp Dijon mustard

1 tsp honey

4 tsp grated Pecorino cheese**

4 tsp fresh basil, finely chopped

crusty, whole grain bread for mopping up sauce

*Rather than using cooking wine, which is pretty terrible stuff, why not use a nice, mid-priced bottle of wine in the stew and serve the rest of the bottle to accompany your aphrodisiac feast?

3. Add the peppers and fennel to the pan and sauté, stirring occasionally, until peppers begin to soften, about 10 minutes.

4. Whisk together the paprika, coriander, salt, pepper, garlic, wine, mustard and honey. Add liquid mixture to the pan and simmer, covered, for 10 minutes.

5. Add grilled sausages to the stew and simmer, uncovered for an additional 5 minutes.

6. Season to taste with salt and pepper—but bear in mind that the cheese will give the dish additional saltiness.

7. To serve, arrange a sausage and 1/4 of the pepper mixture to each plate, making sure to scoop up the liquid. Sprinkle each serving with 1 tsp of the cheese and basil and serve with the crusty, whole grain bread.

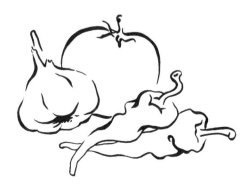

*Little Blue Pill Foods*

# tangerine lemongrass eye-opener mimosas
*makes 2 mimosas*

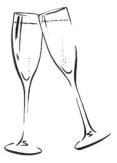

We took the classic brunch drink and dressed it up with a hit of lemongrass, which, in Asian cultures, has been linked with libido. (We just liked the eye-opening, herbal element it added to a very traditional drink.)

1. In each of two Champagne flutes, add 1 tsp lemongrass syrup and 2 oz tangerine or orange-tangerine juice.
2. Top each flute with 3 1/2 or 4 oz chilled Champagne or sparkling wine and serve immediately.

*for the lemongrass syrup:*

1. Add all 3 ingredients to a small saucepan. Bring to a boil then simmer for 30 minutes (depending on the size of your saucepan) or until liquid reduces by 1/2. (If your saucepan is large, keep an eye on the simmering mixture to ensure it doesn't scorch the pan.)
2. Remove from heat and allow syrup to steep until cool.
3. Strain out lemongrass and chill before using.

Leftover syrup can be used as a tangy substitute for simple syrup in any recipe.

2 tsp lemongrass syrup

4 oz tangerine or orange-tangerine juice

7-8 oz Brut Champagne or sparkling wine

*for the lemongrass syrup:*

2 stalks lemongrass, cut into 2″ sections

1/4 c granulated sugar

1/2 c water

# until dawn citrus-coconut water cocktail

*makes 1 cocktail*

The original thought behind this drink was to use coconut water's hydrating properties in a sexy cocktail. We figured it could work as a hangover cure before you ever get the hangover. We called it Until Dawn because it gives you the energy to dance from dusk till dawn!

1 1/2 oz Rémy Martin V.S.O.P.

1/3 c coconut water

1 1/4 tsp simple syrup

1 tsp freshly squeezed calamansi juice**

1 wedge calamansi or tangerine

1 sprig fresh mint

**If you can't find calamansi (a tart, Asian citrus), substitute 1 tsp tangerine juice and 1/4 tsp lemon juice.

1. Combine the Rémy, coconut water, simple syrup and calamansi. Serve, stirred, on the rocks.

2. Garnish with the wedge of fruit and sprig of mint.

*for the simple syrup*

1. To make a simple syrup, bring 1/2 c water to a simmer, add 1/2 c granulated sugar. Stir until sugar dissolves and chill before using. Store leftover syrup in the refrigerator.

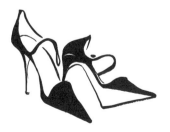

*Little Blue Pill Foods*

# pistachio affogato
vegetarian
*makes 2 servings*

Affogato is an Italian zinger of a dessert. Traditionally it is made with vanilla gelato. But why go Plain Jane when you can serve up a surprising flavor sensation? The combination of steaming hot coffee with ice cream is goose bump-inducing. A wake up call in a glass, the shot of espresso at the end of the meal will have you skipping off to the bedroom, if you even make it that far!

1. Drop 1/3 cup gelato into each of the two servings of espresso. Serve immediately and make magic.

2/3 c pistachio gelato
2 double espresso*

*If you don't have an espresso machine and you love espresso, make the investment. (Ultimately, it is going to save you money over daily coffee bar runs.) But until you can make espresso at home, you have 2 options. Either make the strongest possible coffee using your regular method or pick up coffee from your local haunt and race it home while its still hot. Either way, you'll have something very sexy to serve your sweet.

You can, of course, also try a traditional vanilla bean or chocolate affogato using the proportions above. To take the dish to new aphrodisiac heights, top each serving with a pinch of ground cinnamon.

# 7
# Cook Me Sexy
## *(lower calorie foods)*

If you're looking to shed a few pounds, this chapter is your wheelhouse. While the entire book has focused on delivering a varied diet of nutrient-rich foods, here we've also lowered fat, cholesterol and calories. But we promise you one thing—these recipes don't taste like "diet foods." Instead of making low-cal, low-flavor imitations of comfort food, we've reinterpreted and modernized, as well as lightened up classic dishes. We like to think the result offers new flavor sensations and we know that our slim-down recipes are vitamin rich and will give your libido a delicious little kick.

# wake & bake

vegetarian

*makes 4 servings*

We love breakfast foods. But what we don't love is the crawling out of bed to chop, sauté and stir so we can lavish a lover with a tray of breakfast treats. So we created the Wake and Bake, an aphrodisiac breakfast that can be prepped up to 24 hours in advance. You just go from fridge to oven and hop back in bed to keep someone warm until your breakfast has baked.

1. Coat a nonstick pan with cooking spray. Over medium heat, sauté zucchini, bell pepper, shallot, garlic, oregano and 1/4 tsp salt for 3–4 minutes, until zucchini is soft and shallot begin to brown. Remove from heat and stir in lemon zest.

2. In a separate bowl, stir together flour and milk with a whisk until mixture is lump free.

3. Add egg beaters and salt to milk mixture, whisking until thoroughly combined. Gently stir in Brie.

4. Coat an 8x8 baking dish with cooking spray. Spread vegetable mixture in the bottom of the pan. Pour egg mixture over the top. Cover with plastic wrap and hold in the refrigerator. Dish can be kept, refrigerated, overnight.

*to bake:*

5. Preheat oven to 325 degrees.

2 small zucchini, chopped

1 yellow bell pepper, chopped

1 medium shallot, minced

1 clove garlic, minced

1/4 tsp dried oregano

1/2 tsp salt

1 tsp lemon zest

2 tbsp all-purpose flour

3 tbsp milk

1 1/2 c egg beaters or other liquid eggs

2 oz ripe Brie cheese, (rind on), cut into 1/4" pieces

2 tbsp Gruyère cheese, grated, (added during cooking)

6. Bake, uncovered, for 22–25 minutes or until eggs are just set (once you can shake the pan and it doesn't jiggle). (Baking time may take slightly longer in a glass baking dish.)

7. Remove from oven and sprinkle with Gruyère. Put the baking dish under the broiler for an additional 3–4 minutes, until the top has turned golden brown.

8. Cut into squares and serve warm or at room temperature.

*Optional additional ingredients/alterations:* add 1 tsp chopped, fresh chives or 1 tsp chopped, fresh basil to the egg mixture; replace 1 zucchini with 1 yellow squash or 1 c chopped, fresh spinach; add ham, smoked salmon or veggie ham to the eggs; use truffle salt instead of table salt.

If love your carbs in the morning, stack your eggs on a slice of whole grain toast and garnish the plate with seasonal fruit.

# wake & bake huevos
*(a spicy variation on the Wake and Bake)*
vegetarian
*makes 4 servings*

1. Follow instructions for cooking the vegetables but stir in 3 tbsp salsa and the chile powder with the lemon zest.

2. In step 3, use 2 tbsp grated cheddar or jack in place of the Brie.

3. In step 6, eggs will cook slightly longer, 24–28 minutes to bake.

4. In step 7, top with Cheddar or Jack in place of Gruyère.

5. To serve, garnish each egg square with 1 tbsp salsa and 1 tsp light sour cream.

If you'd like some carbs with that, try toasting a couple of all-natural corn tortillas and serve with additional salsa for dipping.

*additional ingredients:*
7 tbsp your favorite salsa, divided
1/2 tsp chile powder
4 tbsp grated sharp Cheddar or Jack cheese, divided
4 tsp light sour cream

*ingredient adjustments:*
omit Brie
omit Gruyère

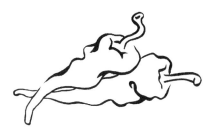

# succulent shrimp
# in a rosemary salt crust
*makes 2 servings*

Roasting shrimp in salt is deceptively easy—frankly, it's almost a parlor trick. Use it for date night since not only will your cooking chops impress but you're serving a dish that has to be eaten with your fingers, (always a sexy experience).

We put this recipe in the "diet" section because it uses a totally fat free, yet exceedingly succulent cooking method. Packing seafood in salt (you can also use this method for roasting whole fish) locks in the moisture but the shell, or in the case of fish, the skin, prevents the sodium from leaching into the meat.

3–4 c coarse salt

4-5 sprigs fresh rosemary

12 jumbo shrimp or prawns, unpeeled*

*You can also use whole prawns with the heads intact. The presentation is a knockout.

1. Preheat oven to 500 degrees.

2. Spread half the salt on the bottom of a baking dish, (8x8 or a small casserole will work).

3. Heat the pan of salt in the oven for 5 minutes. (This will help ensure quick, even cooking.)

4. Lay a bed of rosemary on top of the salt.

5. Arrange shrimp, shells still on, in a single layer on top of the rosemary.

6. Cover with remaining salt.

7. Bake for 10 minutes, then let the dish rest for 2 minutes before removing shrimp from salt and serving warm. (Do not let shrimp rest in salt for more than 5 minutes.)

Serve naked or with your favorite dipping sauce. (Juan-Carlos recommends olive oil with sautéed garlic.)

# grilled chicken spinach salad with plump peaches

*makes 2 servings*

The prep on this recipe couldn't be simpler but the end result is a sweet, salty, crunchy, silky tease to the senses. The salad is at its best on a hot, summer day when peaches are at their peak of freshness. You can try it at other times of the year with each season's finest fruit like apricots in late spring and figs in the fall.

1. Marinate chicken breasts in white wine for 30 minutes to 1 hour, turning once.

2. Brush grill with oil and heat to medium-high heat.

3. Sprinkle each chicken breast with salt and grill for 5 minutes.

4. When the chicken has cooked for 5 minutes, turn to cook for an additional 4–5 minutes and onion slices and peach wedges to the grill.

5. After 2 minutes, flip the onions and peaches.

6. While the chicken is cooking, toss spinach with flax seed oil and divide between two plates. Season with salt and pepper to taste.

7. To serve, top each plate of spinach with a hot chicken breast. Arrange 4 peach wedges and half the onions on each plate. Serve warm.

2 4 oz boneless, skinless chicken breasts

1/2 c dry white wine

olive oil for brushing

1 pinch salt

1/2 medium red onion, sliced into rounds

1 large peach, pitted and sliced into 8 wedges

4 c fresh baby spinach

2 tsp flax seed oil

salt and pepper to taste

# herb-massaged london broil with simple grilled asparagus

*makes 4–6 servings*

In general, we recommend a Love Diet on which beef, a notoriously un-aphrodisiac food, is an indulgence only eaten when you fall off the wagon. Look, if you're about to cry out in protest, face facts. What do you want to do after eating a big steak? Take a big nap, that's what! But if you *must* make red meat a part of your daily life, London Broil is a good choice. It's a cooking method that uses less tender, lower fat cuts of beef (which is why we marinate ours in red wine to tenderize). Then we massage it with herbs to give it at least a hint of aphrodisia. If you like the rub, try using it on anything you like from pork loin to turkey thighs, human thighs... Let your imagination be your guide.

P.S. On our diet, it's ok to fall off the wagon once in awhile. To dine well is human. You just have to have a commitment to get up the next day and climb back aboard the love train.

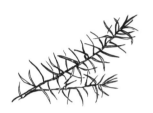

1 c dry red wine

1 top round London Broil, 1 1/4 to 1 1/2 lbs (about 1 1/4" thick)

2 tsp coarse salt

1/2 tsp black pepper

1 tbsp fresh sage, chopped

1 tbsp fresh thyme

2 tbsp fresh rosemary, chopped

1 medium shallot, minced

1 lb asparagus, ends trimmed

salt to taste

1. Trim meat of all visible fat.

2. Let London broil marinate, refrigerated in red wine for 1–2 hours.

3. Remove meat form marinade. Pat dry and transfer to a broiler pan. Allow meat to come to room temperature (about 45 minutes).

4. Combine rub ingredients (2 tsp salt, black pepper, sage, thyme, rosemary and shallot) and thoroughly coat meat.

*Cook Me Sexy*

5. Turn broiler to high and broil meat approximately 8" under the flame for 7–8 minutes per side, turning once, for medium rare to medium doneness.

*for the asparagus:*
1. Coat grill or stove top grill pan with a little cooking oil then heat to medium-high.
2. Cook asparagus for 3–5 minutes depending on thickness, turning once.
3. Remove from grill and season with salt.

Serve with a glass of red wine and roasted sweet potatoes. Or try it with our sweet potato-shallot purée, page 46.

# black truffle lovers' lasagna
vegetarian
*makes 4 servings*

The scent of black truffle is very similar to that of a male pheromone. (Pheromones are human, sexual scents that unconsciously register as attraction in possible mates.) And we know women who swear by as little as a single whiff of truffles as producing the... ahem... desired effect. Because we can't afford to run out and buy black truffles every time we're looking for action, we've created a dish that uses black truffle oil and salt in such a way that it releases that aroma of desire into the air.

1 1/2 c eggplant, chopped

1/2 tsp salt

2 1/2 tsp black truffle-infused oil

1 clove garlic, crushed

1 portabella mushroom cap, minced

2 medium zucchini, chopped

2 c baby spinach salad leaves, roughly chopped

1 tsp black truffle salt

1 tbsp fresh basil, chopped

1 c part skim ricotta

6 no-cook lasagna noodles

1/4 c Parmesan, grated

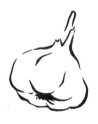

1. Sprinkle the eggplant with the 1/2 tsp salt, set aside for 10 minutes. (Eggplant will discolor slightly.)

2. Preheat oven to 375 degrees, and coat an 8 or 9-inch square baking dish with nonstick cooking spray.

3. Heat oil in a large, nonstick pan over medium heat. Sauté garlic for 1 minute.

4. Add mushroom and sauté for an additional minute.

5. Stir in eggplant and zucchini. Gently sauté for 10 minutes, until vegetables are softened.

6. Stir in spinach and truffle salt then remove from heat when the spinach begins to wilt.

7. Add basil and ricotta and thoroughly mix.

8. Spread 1/4 of the vegetable mixture on the bottom of the baking dish. Top with 2 noodles, followed by 1/4 of the vegetables; then 2 more noodles, repeat, then finish with the last 1/4 of the vegetables.

9. Top with grated Parmesan, cover pan with foil and bake for 20 minutes.

10. Uncover and cook for an additional 5 minutes. For a crunchy top, put under the broiler for an additional 3–5 minutes, until cheese is deep golden.

*Cook Me Sexy*

# summertime limoncello spritzer
*makes 2 servings*

Amy's mom actually invented this cocktail. She wanted to come up with a drink that was refreshing and interesting but low enough in alcohol that it could be enjoyed all day long. Using Limoncello is a great call because not only is it sweet, tart and fresh but offers flavors strong enough to carry a cocktail on its own, making the drink low alcohol and low-cal. You can shake and strain it if you don't like the muddled mint in your glass but we prefer the simplicity of the method below.

1. Muddle 2 sprig of mint at the bottom of 2 rocks glasses.

2. Divide ice and Limoncello between the 2 glasses.

3. Top with club soda and garnish with remaining mint.

4 sprigs fresh mint
6 fresh ice cubes*
3 oz Limoncello
club soda

*Ice quickly takes on a freezer taste and you don't want a cocktail with a flavor of freezer burn. Throw out unused ice frequently to ensure a fresh flavor.

# chocolate mint seduction cookies

vegetarian

*makes approximately 24 cookies*

1 c all-purpose flour

1/4 tsp baking soda

1/4 tsp salt

1/2 c high-fat cocoa powder, sifted*

4 tbsp butter, softened

1/2 c brown sugar, packed

1/2 c granulated sugar

3 tbsp unsweetened applesauce

3/4 tsp vanilla extract

1 large egg white, at room temperature, fork beaten

3/4 c mini Andes Candies or regular Andes Candies, chopped into pieces approximately the size of mini chocolate chips

*Premium cocoa powders have a higher percentage of cocoa powder, which translates in flavor to a far richer, chocolate taste. Of the premium brands, we like Callebaut. For a lower-priced option, try Hershey's Special Dark.

I came up with this recipe several years ago looking to create something with Christmas flavors that wasn't based on butter. The trick, I discovered, was to keep some of the fat, which gives cookies their crisp texture. The final recipe uses applesauce to replace some (but not all) of the butter and then uses egg white for volume and texture. The combination of high-fat cocoa powder and mint makes the cookie satisfying and refreshing all at once. It is definitely the lightest Christmas cookie I've ever made. My thighs have thanked me for years!—Amy

1. Combine flour, baking soda, salt and cocoa in a small mixing bowl. Set aside.

2. In a mixing bowl, stir butter until creamy. Add the sugars and mix until combined, about 1 minute by hand. Then add applesauce and vanilla, stirring to combine.

3. Add the egg white to the sugar mixture and beat for an additional 1–2 minutes.

4. Add the flour mixture, stirring until thoroughly combined. (The dough will be fairly stiff.)

5. Fold in the Andes Candies pieces.

6. Coat your hands lightly with oil and shape the cookie dough into 2 5" logs. Wrap logs in plastic wrap and freeze 1–2 hours or until firm.

*Cook Me Sexy*

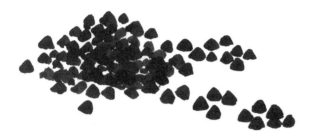

7.  Preheat oven to 350 degrees.

8.  Coat baking sheet(s) with cooking spray.

9.  Unwrap frozen logs and slice into approximately 24 rounds, (about 1/4" thick). Place the rounds on the baking sheet 1" apart.

10. Bake on the center rack for 8–9 minutes then remove from sheet and allow to cool. (If cookies are difficult to remove from the sheet, allow them to cool on the sheet for 30 seconds before removing.)

11. Eat.

# individual phyllo fruit tarts with smoked salt

vegetarian

*makes 4 tarts*

You can make these tarts up to 2 days in advance, which makes them about our handiest dessert. And because they are made with phyllo and fresh fruit, they're healthy and low-fat but in our taste tests they've proven to satisfy the whole family. As an aphrodisiac, the ginger can help raise body temperature. But it's the unique addition of smoked salt that sets our tarts apart. So be sure, though you might be tempted, not to skip this step. The sensations of smoky and savory tease your mouth with a new, goose bump-worthy flavor sensation. Now *that's* the mark of a good tart!

2 tsp butter

3 c apples or peaches, peeled, cored and thinly sliced

2 tbsp and 2 tsp granulated sugar

1 tsp lemon juice

1/4 c apple or white grape juice

1 tbsp candied ginger, finely chopped

1/4 tsp cinnamon

4 sheets phyllo dough, thawed

1/4 tsp smoked salt*

*Smoked salt can be found at specialty gourmet retailers and online.

1. Melt butter in a nonstick sauté pan over medium heat.

2. Add apples or peaches and 1 tsp sugar. Sauté 5 minutes or until lightly browned. Remove from heat and stir in lemon juice. Allow fruit to cool slightly.

3. In a small saucepan, heat white grape or apple juice, candied ginger and 2 tbsp sugar, stirring until sugar is dissolved.

4. In a small bowl, mix together the remaining tsp sugar with the cinnamon.

5. Coat 4 individual (4-oz) ramekins with cooking spray. (If you don't own ramekins, you can use sturdy coffee mugs.)

*Cook Me Sexy*

6. Take one sheet of phyllo, spray lightly with cooking spray and sprinkle with 1/4 of the sugar mixture.

7. Fold phyllo in half, then quarters, and gently shape it into the bottom of a ramekin so that extra dough is hanging over the edges.

8. Spray it again with the cooking spray.

9. Fill with 1/4 of the cooked fruit and 1/4 of the syrup. Top each with 1/4 of the smoked salt. With damp fingers, gently fold the overhanging phyllo to cover the fruit, making a top crust. Repeat with three remaining ramekins.

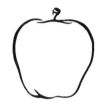

10. Cover tightly with plastic wrap and store in the refrigerator until you are ready to bake. Uncooked tarts can keep, refrigerated, for up to 48 hours.

*to bake:*

1. Preheat oven to 350 degrees.

2. Cook each ramekin on the middle rack for 20 minutes or until edges of phyllo crust are a deep, golden brown. Cool a few minutes before serving.

# 8
# Nibbles, Snacks and a Little Something on the Side

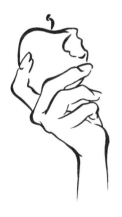

We've said it before: We are both snackers. And we speak from personal experience when we say that allowing too much time to pass between meals can result in gorging on everything in sight, (followed by heavy doses of guilt and none-too-sexy bloating). Snacks will keep your blood sugar steady and can hold cravings at bay. In this chapter, we're sharing some of our favorite snacks for keeping mind and body on an even keel and libido levels at a climax.

# bikini bread

vegetarian

*makes 1 loaf*

As a child, I thought a two-piece bathing suit was called a zucchini. Even though I no longer confuse my bikini with a summer squash, I still think the two have something in common. Made with whole wheat flour, a dose of veggies and healthy walnuts, this sweet can actually help keep you in bikini shape. I like to serve bikini bread as an alternative to a muffin or scone or as a pick-me-up for the afternoon slump.—Amy

1. Preheat oven to 350 degrees (325 degrees if using a glass loaf pan).

2. Sift together flour, salt, baking soda, baking powder and cinnamon. Set aside.

3. Using an electric mixer, beat eggs on medium speed for 2 minutes.

4. Add sugar, oil and vanilla and beat for an additional 2 minutes then mix in zucchini.

5. Turn mixer speed to low and add in the flour mixture, about 1/2 cup at a time, mixing until flour is just combined. Fold in walnuts (optional).*

6. Pour batter into a loaf pan that has been thoroughly greased and floured and bake until an inserted toothpick or cake tester comes out clean, about 45–55 minutes.

7. Remove from pan immediately and cool on wire rack.

1 1/2 c whole wheat flour

1/2 tsp salt

1/4 tsp baking soda

1/4 tsp baking powder

2 tsp cinnamon

2 eggs, room temperature

1 c sugar

1/2 c vegetable oil

1 1/2 tsp vanilla

1 c zucchini, grated

1/2 chopped walnuts, (optional)

*Batter can be made up to 24 hours in advance.

# black olives with basil confetti

vegetarian

*makes 4 servings*

Paired with a glass of dry rosé wine, this is the perfect appetizer for a hot, summer evening. Olives are one of those foods you get to play with, which earns them high marks in our books. The preparation of this summer snack is insanely simple and the herbal element of the basil makes salty olives suddenly refreshing.

24 black olives with pits, (such as kalamata)*

1 tbsp fresh basil leaves

*Experiment with the gourmet olive selection at your grocery store or local gourmet food store. You will discover there is a whole world of delicious, uniquely different olives out there from those sliced black specks on salad bars.

1. Place the olives in a serving dish.

2. Stack the basil leaves and roll them lengthwise. Using a sharp pairing knife, slice the roll into thin segments to make ribbons. Sprinkle over the olives and serve.

# surprise someone soybean dip

vegetarian

*makes 4 servings*

You typically see soybeans (edamame) in Japanese restaurants, ( those little snacks served in the pod). But you can also buy shelled soybeans in the freezer section of many grocery and health food stores. Keep a bag handy to make this quick dip for last minute guests, or as a light snack on nights when you're too tired to cook. You can also use it as a sandwich spread (see open-faced grilled cheese below) or serve it to your kids with a bowl of chips to sneak some veggies into their diets. No one will believe that this dip is made from soybeans–or that it's full of fantastic nutrients.

*Nibbles, Snacks*

1. Put ingredients in a blender and purée until smooth.

2. Season with salt and pepper before serving.

3. Serve as a dip with vegetables, chips or thyme-sprinkled whole wheat pita chips (page 113), or use as a spread on sandwiches.

   Dip can be kept, refrigerated, for up to 5 days.

1 c steamed soybeans (edamame)

1/4 c fresh spinach leaves, roughly chopped

1/4 tsp garlic, (approx 1/2 clove), minced

1 tbsp lemon juice

2 tsp olive oil

1/2 c vegetable stock

1/2 tsp dry mustard

salt and white pepper to taste

# open-faced grilled cheese with soybean dip
*makes 1 sandwich*

1. Spread both sides of the bread with a thin layer of butter.

2. Heat a nonstick pan over medium heat. Toast one side of the bread to golden brown, flip the bread and remove it from the pan.

3. Spread the toasted side of the bread with the soybean dip and sprinkle with the cheese.

4. Return the sandwich to the pan, uncooked side down and cook to a golden brown.

5. Put the sandwich under the broiler until the cheese starts to bubble.

1 slice your favorite sandwich bread

1-2 tsp butter

1 tbsp soybean dip, (above)

2 tbsp your favorite cheese, grated

# thyme-sprinkled
# whole wheat pita chips
*makes 4 servings*

This is our quick and simple alternative to the ultra processed crunchy things sold in the grocery store snack aisle. We think that the thyme leaves combined with earthy, whole wheat take snacking to a new level. Try them with anything from our soy dip (page 111), to guacamole, goat's milk cheese and even tomato-anchovy bruschetta (page 60).

2 whole wheat pitas
olive oil for brushing
2 tsp fresh thyme
leaves

1. Preheat oven to 350 degrees.

2. Using a pastry brush, brush both sides of each pita with olive oil.

3. Sprinkle the tops of the pitas with the thyme leaves, pressing them down slightly, into the oil.*

4. Cut each pita into 6 triangles and arrange the triangles on a baking sheet.

5. Bake until the pitas crisp, 12–16 minutes, depending on your oven and the thickness of the pitas. (If you like your pitas crisp on the edges with softness in the middle, cook for a shorter period of time. If you like them completely crunchy, cook longer but check frequently to avoid burning.)

\* If you like your snacks a little salty, you can sprinkle the tops with a pinch of coarse sea salt when you add the thyme.

*Nibbles, Snacks*

# one & only salad dressing

*makes 4-6 servings*

Not only is this the perfect dressing for your one and only but this is the one and only vinaigrette I make! I change it up a little every time. Sometimes I add a little balsamic vinegar and sometimes a pinch of Herbes de Provence. The reason that we've deemed it the perfect Love Diet salad dressing is that it uses only enough oil to cling to the lettuce leaves and such intensity of flavor that you need only use a low-calorie little splash.—Amy

1. Finely mince shallot and put it, along with the red wine vinegar, Dijon and rosemary into a small mixing bowl,

2. Using a wire whisk, slowly whisk in the olive oil, using just enough to give the dressing a glossy shine and vinaigrette consistency.

3. Season with salt and pepper to taste.

1/2 medium shallot

2 tbsp red wine vinegar

1 tbsp Dijon mustard

1 pinch dried rosemary

1–2 tsp fruity olive oil

salt and pepper to taste

# feta & basil stuffed mushrooms

vegetarian

*makes 4 servings*

Nobody will ever guess that the stuffing in these mushrooms is half tofu. The thing about tofu is that it tends to take on the flavor of whatever is cooked with it, so here, the tofu pretty much tastes like feta. But you're still getting all of tofu's health benefits, including its low-calorie protein and estrogen.

12 large or "stuffing" white mushrooms caps

1 tsp olive oil

1/4 c yellow onion, finely chopped

1 garlic clove, minced

1/2 c light tofu

1/4 tsp mustard powder

1 tsp Worcestershire sauce

1/4 tsp salt

1/4 tsp black pepper

1/3 c fat free feta

1/4 c fresh baby spinach, roughly chopped

1 tbsp fresh basil, minced

2 tbsp panko, (Japanese breadcrumbs)

1. Preheat oven to 350 degrees.

2. Wash mushrooms and remove stems. Place mushrooms stem-side down in a shallow baking dish coated with cooking spray. Cook for 10 minutes. Remove any excess liquid from the baking dish and set aside.

3. In a nonstick sauté pan, heat olive oil. Sauté the onions until soft, about 2 minutes. Add in garlic, tofu, mustard powder, Worcestershire sauce, salt and pepper and cook for an additional 2 minutes.

4. Add in feta, spinach and basil and remove pan from heat.

5. Stir in panko.

6. Turn mushrooms over so that the stuffing side is up then stuff the mushrooms.

7. Cook for 15 minutes or until mushrooms are tender and stuffing has turned slightly golden.

*Nibbles, Snacks*

# simple roasted vegetables
*serves 4 as a side or 2 as a main course*

We don't deny it, we both love cheese (which is a proven aphrodisiac). And we've found that cheese is one thing that can get just about anyone to eat their vegetables. We use just a touch, to keep the fat content low, but the flavor does deliver. We've been able to coax many a veggie hater to eat this dish. (If you aren't trying to lose weight or watch your cholesterol, you can double the cheese for a really powerful flavor. This works particularly well in enticing kids—and those with palates of children.)

1. Preheat oven to 375 degrees.

2. Cut the leek in half lengthwise then thoroughly wash. Chop white part through the first 2" of green into 1/4" half-circles, discarding dark greens. (The dark leaves can be reserved and used to flavor a vegetable stock.)

3. Chop the 2 cups of vegetables into bite-sized pieces.

4. In a shallow baking dish that has been coated with nonstick cooking spray, combine leeks and other vegetables with the oil, garlic, salt and pepper.

5. Bake, covered, for 20 minutes. Stir, then cook uncovered for an additional 10-15 minutes until vegetables are fork-tender.

1 leek

2 c any combination of brussel sprouts, zucchini, yellow squash, wax beans, cauliflower, broccolini

1 tbsp olive oil

1 tsp garlic, finely minced

1/4 tsp salt

1/4 tsp pepper

2 Tbsp hard cheese of choice, such as Parmesan, Pecorino, Gruyère or aged Jack, grated

6. Top baked vegetables with cheese and heat under broiler until cheese browns, about 3 minutes.

Serve with your favorite main course or as a light meal, accompanied by whole grain bread and butter.

*Optional additional ingredients/alterations:* add 1 tbsp basil or thyme or 1 tbsp balsamic, red wine vinegar or lemon juice to the vegetable mixture; add 1/2 c chopped mushrooms; toss with butter instead of oil; sprinkle baked vegetables with parsley or chives.

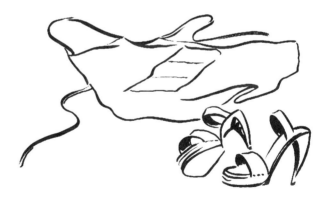

# blue cheese walnut brittle

vegetarian

*makes 12-14 servings*

From the title, this recipe may sound like one our craziest ideas; and it is. But it makes one of the most interesting dishes in this book. We love the earthy flavor that the aphrodisiac walnuts, thyme and blue cheese add to what is often an overly-sweet snack. Most brittle recipes start with water and allow it to evaporate through the cooking process. Juan-Carlos' method for making brittle is much simpler and quicker—the sugar simply melts in the pan like magic, although the process requires faithful attention. Making this recipe is incredibly fun, just be careful when working with hot sugar. One touch can cause a painful burn.

1. Chop the thyme leaves to release some of their oil.

2. In a small mixing bowl, toss together the walnuts, blue cheese and thyme until walnuts are thoroughly coated with cheese and no visible blue cheese crumbles remain. Set aside.

3. Line a baking sheet with wax paper or, ideally, a silicone baking mat. If using wax paper, brush the surface of the wax paper with oil. Lay an identical-sized piece of wax paper (or silicone mat) on the counter and brush with oil.

4. Heat a heavy saucepan over high heat. When pan is hot, sprinkle in just enough of the sugar to coat the bottom of the pan and begin to stir the sugar. Sugar will start to melt into a caramel.

1 tsp fresh thyme leaves

1 1/4 c roasted, unsalted walnuts, coarsely chopped*

1/4 c blue cheese, crumbled

oil for brushing

2 c granulated sugar

1/2 tsp coarse salt

*Unsalted walnuts can be found in the baking section of most grocery stores. Look for "baking pieces" to get a pre-chopped product.

5. Turn temperature down to medium and sprinkle in more sugar, 3 tbsp at a time, stirring. Continue adding sugar at this rate as the hot sugar melts. If the color of the mixture starts to get any darker than light amber, remove the pan from the heat for a few seconds to allow it to cool.

6. Once you've used half of the sugar, begin adding sugar to the mixture at a rate of 1/3 cup at a time. Continue to stir and monitor the color. You do not want the sugar to get too dark.

7. When all the sugar has been incorporated, turn heat to low and add the walnut mixture, stirring until incorporated.

8. Quickly transfer brittle from the pan to the lined baking sheet. Be careful not to touch the hot brittle, it will burn. Cover the brittle with the second sheet of wax paper (oil side down) or silicone mat. Using a rolling pin, roll brittle out to about a 1/4" to 1/3" thickness.

9. Allow brittle to cool for about 5-8 minutes, until top layer of wax paper pulls back easily, but surface of the brittle is still a little sticky. Sprinkle the top with the salt then allow the brittle to cool completely before removing from the tray and breaking into pieces.

Store brittle in an airtight container.

# bedtime yogurt

vegetarian

*makes 4 servings*

As we've mentioned, we believe in the healing power of a bedtime snack. The trick is finding a snack that satisfies but doesn't spend the night traveling from lip to hip. This is one of our go-to nighttime snacks because it offers protein without a whole lot of unwanted sugar, fat or additives. In season, you can use fresh strawberries but with frozen, you can enjoy the snack year-round.

1. In a small saucepan, combine strawberries, brown rice syrup or agave nectar and water.

2. Bring to a simmer over medium-low heat, stirring occasionally.

Once mixture starts to simmer, turn the heat to low and allow strawberries to cook for 10-15 minutes until mixture resembles a loose jam.

3. Cool completely and store in the refrigerator.

4. Spoon 1/4 of the cooled strawberry mixture over each of 4 1/2 cup servings of yogurt.

For a variation, try using 1/2 cup strawberries and 1/2 cup rhubarb.

1 c frozen strawberries, roughly chopped

2 tbsp brown rice syrup or 1 tbsp agave nectar*

1/4 c water

2 c plain, Greek-style yogurt

*We recommend brown rice syrup and agave, both found at health food retailers, because they don't cause the blood sugar spike of refined sugar. You can also use either white or brown sugar if you prefer but be careful that it doesn't keep you awake.

# Dictionary of Desire

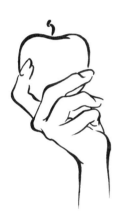 There is no doubt that certain ingredients will help your experience in the bedroom. However, in many cases, the amount of an ingredient required to set the bed alight has yet to be fully researched. The goal of this book is to get you eating a broad range of foods that will make your mind and body positively sing. We know you aren't always going to be able to eat from the recipes in this book, so we've detailed some of the foods and nutrients that make smart choices when you're dining out, on the run or just trying something new.

**Foods of Desire**—*Some of our favorite aphrodisiac foods include, but are not limited to:*

*Apples*—The symbol of temptation—and of health— apples are the true emblem of the aphrodisiac world. But apples' powers of temptation are not in the looks department alone. Their antioxidants fight aging and the fruit's skin offers much-needed fiber. (An aphrodisiac truth: regularity can be one of the keys to a happy relationship!)

*Blueberries*—Low in calories and high in fiber, blueberries have one of the highest antioxidant levels among all fruits. And, according to health professor Mary Ellen Carnire, their nutritional makeup can also help to alleviate erectile malfunctions.

*Buffalo—see Wild Game*

*Champagne (and other sparkling wines)*—Champagne not only offers the heart health benefits of red wine but studies show that sparkling wine can be helpful in preventing brain deterioration. From personal experience, we also maintain that bubbly brings an air of flirtation and festivity to any occasion and that the pearl-like strings bubbles hitting the bloodstream results in giddy abandon. Salud!

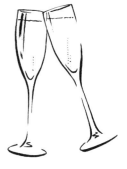

*Cheese*—Doctors say that cheese is great for the teeth because it lowers levels of bacteria in the mouth. Makes you want to kiss a cheese eater, doesn't it? Cheese also contains phenylethylamine, a naturally-occurring chemical compound that acts as a sort of natural amphetamine. Researcher Dr. Max Lake found that the scent of triple cream cheeses replicated that of a female pheromone. (Who would have thought brie could bring excitement to your bedroom?) Just remember that although cheese is definitely a Love Diet do, too much of a good thing can sometimes find you fat and alone.

*Chile Peppers*—One of the most talked-about aphrodisiacs of the plant world, chile has the ability to raise body temperature, make the tongue tingle and bring an alluring flush to the cheeks. Some researchers have even said that eating chiles can cause an all-out endorphin rush. (We don't know about you but we think this sounds much more appealing than running a marathon for that natural high.)

*Chocolate*—It *is* true that chocolate contains chemical compounds with the potential for elevating mood, perking energy and warming things in the nether regions. But—we hate to break it to you—its been proven that an average-sized adult would have to consume more than 20 lbs of chocolate in one sitting to achieve such a hot rush. *(Diabetic coma, anyone?)* That being said, chocolate's caffeine-like properties can boost energy and the antioxidants in dark chocolate and cocoa can be beneficial in the fight against aging.

*Cocoa—see Chocolate*

*Coffee*—The aphrodisiac of adrenalin, coffee is an excellent aid for sparking amorous encounters. Coffee can also rev up metabolism and its been shown to aid concentration. Scientific studies have even proved that coffee can promote the production of dopamine, a neurotransmitter associated not only with pleasure but also cognition, memory and motivation.

*Garlic*—Garlic is a global cure-all as old as recorded time. It has been used to treat everything from sleep apnea to cancer. The Ancient Greeks fed it to their athletes prior to Olympic competition for increased stamina—the kind of assistance we could all use, be we Olympians or common folk.

*Ginger*—Ginger is fantastic for warming up the body and the bedroom. It is effective in stimulating both the circulatory and digestive systems. We want that blood pumping!

*Honey*—An all-natural sweetener, honey is sexy just in its appearance (and the promise of playtime a little drizzle can spark). But it also offers the body boron, which helps us utilize estrogen. And, of course, a little taste can boost blood sugar and offer a bit of energy at a critical moment.

*Mussels*—In 2005, a group of researchers discovered that an amino acid in mussels directly raised sexual hormone levels—how's that for an aphrodisiac? A lean protein, mussels are also a good mood food, providing Omega-3's.

*Mustard*—We think of mustard as that yellow paste

smeared on ham sandwiches, but mustard seed is actually a sexual powerhouse rich in aphrodisiac history. Until modern times, monks were banned from eating mustard because of its aphrodisiac powers. Today, we know that mustard seeds offer several nutrients vital to sexual health, including selenium, magnesium, Omega-3's and zinc.

*Nuts*—Nuts are high in fiber and protein. They provide the body with vitamin E, also called the "sex vitamin." In addition, studies indicate that nuts have the potential to elevate serotonin levels, a bonus, feel-good effect.

*Oysters*—The old cliché is true, oysters are great for your sex life (unless you're allergic to bivalves). Yes, they're a good source of zinc and lean protein but thanks to recent research, we suspect that they could also promote sexual hormone production.

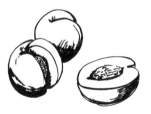

*Peaches*—Sweet, fuzzy peaches earned a folkloric rep as aphrodisiacs because, it was felt, their form resembled a curvaceous, female buttock. We're not so sure about the comparison but we do know that peaches are a good source of fiber, vitamin C, vitamin A and also offer some potassium and magnesium.

*Salmon*—Not only is the pink fish known as one of the best sources of mood-enhancing Omega-3's, it offers calcium and vitamin A. (You knew anything that pretty on a plate had to be great for something!)

*Dictionary of Desire*

*Scallops*—Scallops probably first earned their aphrodisiac reputation for their voluptuous, sexy, slippery mouthfeel—a little bit of naughty on the tongue. We now know that scallops provide lean protein and iodine and may, according to the findings of a recent study, contain an amino acid that raises sexual hormone levels.

*Shrimp*—Shrimp offer lean protein (as in, it supplies energy all night long), iodine, Omega-3's, iron and zinc. What's not to love? *(We recommend buying wild caught shrimp, as farming practices in some countries use chemicals that can be harmful to both your health and the environment.)*

*Soybeans*—Soy is a sensational source of protein and, as such, can increases dopamine. It contains plant estrogens and has been helpful in relieving PMS and menopausal symptoms like vaginal dryness. There is also some evidence that soy is beneficial to prostate health.

*Sparkling Wine—see Champagne*

*Spinach and other dark leafies*—You may never have thought "spinach" and "sex" in the same sentence but dark leafy greens have got it going on in ways that will get *you* going in the bedroom. Low in calories, sans fat, spinach offers magnesium, as well as a dose of vitamins A and C. Kale, another one of the dark leafies, is off the charts in terms of vitamin A.

*Tofu—see Soybeans*

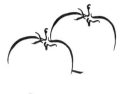

*Tomatoes*—Sexy, scarlet red tomatoes bring not only the color of love to the plate, but offer lycopene, beneficial to prostate health. Tomatoes are also a source of vitamins A and C.

*Truffles*—One for the ladies, the musky scent of truffles is said to smell almost identical to androstenone, a male pheromone. Truffle cologne, anyone?

*Watermelon*—It was recently discovered that one of watermelon's phytonutrients, citrulline, can relax blood vessels, acting as a natural Viagra. It is also an excellent source of lycopine, beneficial to prostate health.

*Whole Grains*—You know the saying that people on a diet should stay away from "white things"? Well, people on The Love Diet should trade in that white for as many whole grains as possible for beneficial B vitamins and fiber. You're lover will thank us later.

*Wild Game*—If you enjoy red meat, try wild game like buffalo, venison, wild boar, pheasant and antelope. (Farmed buffalo, venison and duck are also great choices.) Leaner than beef and lamb, wild game meats can increases dopamine and norepinephrine production in the brain and provide sustained energy without a lot of saturated fat. Besides, serving something *wild* can make you feel like you're living on the edge!

*Dictionary of Desire*

*Wine*—Some experts say that a glass a day could keep the doctor away. We now know that red wine and Champagne offer powerful antioxidants. Some research has shown that the aromas of wines can replicate human pheromones. More obviously, we know that a little wine can lower inhibition and take the edge off during a romantic encounter. But, of course, always keep in mind that too much wine can turn a pas de deux into a *snore for you*!

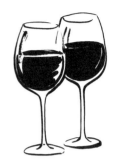

*Yogurt*—Slathering yourself in yogurt may not make you more sexy, but eating this fantastic food will provide you with protein and calcium not to mention B vitamins and magnesium. And by the way, we do hear that a yogurt face mask can give your skin a certain glow.

**Nutrients for Nakedness**

We've detailed these nutrients with foods that are recommended sources. Should you decide to up your intake of any of these nutrients via vitamins and supplements, we recommend consulting your physician for individualized dosage instructions.

*B Vitamins*—Vitamin B deficiencies only became common in the Western diet after the invention of white bread. (Gee, thanks Wonder Bread!) The B's fight depression, elevate energy and mood, promote bloodflow and fight stress. We all need to make every effort possible to get our B's with foods like: **whole**

**wheat; brewer's yeast; dairy; beans; seeds** and **dark, leafy greens**.

*Essential Fatty Acids*—If you thought "fat" was a four-letter word, count again. Essential fatty acids not only promote muscle growth but they're needed for the production of sex hormones and can improve circulation (the better the blood pumps, the better the orgasm). Sources include: **sunflower** and **sesame oils; walnuts; peanut butter** (for linoleic acid) and **salmon; sardines; anchovies** and **flax seed oil** (for Omega-3's).

*Iodine*—This mineral is essential to the thyroid gland. Without ample iodine, you may feel reduced sex drive and low energy. If you use iodized salt, you're already supplementing your diet, but other sources include: **seafoods; yogurt; eggs** and **pineapple**.

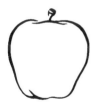

*Magnesium*—Research has proven that this mineral is absolutely essential to sex hormone production. It can also help reduce muscle soreness and cramps and can, shall we say, give your colon a call to action. (Face it, bowel issues are a hazard to your sex life.) To increase magnesium intake, try: **soybeans; apples; bananas; figs** and **dairy products**.

*Manganese*—A key ingredient in eating for your sex life, manganese not only fights free radicals to prevent premature aging, but in a lab study, manganese-deficient male animals had a lack of semen and—scary—degeneration of the seminal tubules.

*Dictionary of Desire*

Boys, eat your **leafy greens; nuts; berries; whole grains** and **coffee**.

*Selenium*—Did you know that sperm is loaded with selenium? Therefore, anyone involved with a selenium-deficient man is in trouble! Selenium is also known to boost mood and slow the aging process. Get your selenium from **onions; garlic; poultry; whole grains** and **mushrooms**.

*Vitamin A*—Some nutrients require each other to support you. Vitamin A supports vitamin E in promoting sperm production. It is also essential for a healthy thyroid. To make your vitamin A intake an A +, try **milk; yams; pumpkin; eggs; tomatoes** and **leafy greens**.

*Vitamin C*—Vitamin C is a major supporter of the adrenal glands. Bluntly put, you can't have an orgasm without vitamin C. Now go eat an orange. Vitamin C is also great for the immune system and can help keep your joints limber. Besides citrus, sources of C include **strawberries; kale; bell peppers; papaya** and **broccoli**.

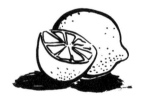

*Vitamin E*—Many people call it the "sex vitamin." Vitamin E is required for the production of sexual hormones and can help increase a low sperm count. It also offers antioxidant powers to keep you young and sexy. We know some of you are thinking you already have an E that is great for your sex life but get enough of your vitamins and *this* is the only E you need. For

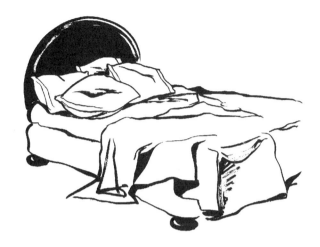

better sex the natural way, try **nuts; seeds; eggs; mangos; spinach** and **asparagus**.

*Zinc*—The "man's mineral," zinc promotes blood flow to the family jewels, aids in testosterone production and is essential for prostate health. Eat up boys: **oysters; pumpkin seeds; yogurt** and **whole grains**.

# *Select References*

Abend, Lisa. "How Cows (Grass-Fed Only) Could Save the Planet." *Time* January 25, 2010. Web. February 20, 2010. <http://www.time.com/time/magazine/article/0,9171,1953692,00.html>.

Albertson, Ellen and Michael Albertson. *Temptations: igniting the pleasure and power of aphrodisiacs.* New York: Fireside, 2002.

"Dictionary of Aphrodisiac Foods." Eat Something Sexy. Web. January 5, 2010. <http://www.eatsome-thingsexy.com/aphrodisiac/index.htm>.

Gaffney, Jacob. "Pop the Champagne for Heart Health." *Wine Spectator* December 9, 2009. Web. December 12, 2009. <http://www.winespectator.com/webfeature/show/id/41383>.

"Health Impacts." Food & Water Watch December 12, 2009. Web. February 10, 2010. < http://www.food andwaterwatch.org/fish/fish-farming/shrimp/ health-impacts/>.

Hirsch M.D., Alan R. *Scentsational Sex.* Boston: Element Books, Inc., 1998.

Lake M.D., Max. *Scents and Sesuality.* London: Futura, 1989.

Lawlis, Dr. Frank and Dr. Maggie Greenwood-Robin-son. *The Brain Power Cookbook.* New York: Penguin Books, 2009.

Liebowitz M.D., Michael R. *The Chemistry of Love.* New York: Little, Brown, 1983.

McCullough, Marie. "Coffee's Health Conundrums." *The Seattle Times* July 30, 2006. Web. February 6, 2010. <http://seattletimes.nwsource.com/ html/health/2003159425_healthcoffee30.html>

Mervis Watson M.D., Cynthia. *Love Potions.* Los Ange-les: Tarcher/Perigee, 1993.

Nickel, Nancy L. *Nature's Aphrodisiacs*. Freedom, CA: The Crossing Press, 2001.

Pollan, Michael. *The Omnivore's Dilemma*. New York: Penguin Books, 2006.

Rolls Ph.D., Barbara. *The Volumetrics Eating Plan*. New York: Harper Collins, 2004.

# Index

*Index*

# About the Authors

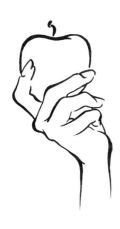

**Juan-Carlos Cruz** is best known as the host of the two Food Network shows, "Calorie Commando" and "Weighing In," as well as host of Discovery Health Network's "Body Challenge 3." Cruz formally trained at the California Culinary Academy and has worked as a pastry chef in hotels and restaurants, including the illustrious Hotel Bel Air.

Clearly a fan of his own work, Cruz packed on 100 lbs during his years of baking. After very publicly losing 43 lbs of it on Discovery's "Body Challenge 1," the self-described recovering pastry chef changed his culinary style from sweet tooth to veggie pusher and launched Calorie Commando Catering.

Evidently, Cruz's catering business hit a nerve with the American public, as it quickly led to projects with the Food Network, American Heart Association and Cruz's first book, *The Calorie Countdown Cookbook.*

Most recently Cruz has broadened his goal, in collaboration with Amy Reiley, to help home cooks get fit, happy and frisky in and out of the kitchen. Cruz shares a home with his wife Jennifer, who remains frisky after more than 20 years of marriage, and their two "kids," Norwich Terriers Maggie and Nick.

**Amy Reiley** has been recognized as a leading authority on aphrodisiac foods by publications as varied as National Geographic and The London Times. Creator of EatSomethingSexy.com, as well as author of *Fork Me, Spoon Me:* the sensual cookbook, she was the second American to earn a Master's Degree in Gastronomy from Le Cordon Bleu.

Reiley has appeared as an aphrodisiacs expert on television and radio programs from "The CBS Early Show" to NPR's "Wait Wait...Don't Tell Me!" She has also appeared on Playboy television—you'll recognize her as the one wearing clothing.

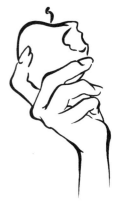

In addition to her quirky niche, Reiley is noted as an internationally published wine journalist and critic. She consults with wineries and restaurants on pairings, cocktail development and aphrodisiac-inspired events. Reiley travels, teaching and speaking on food, wine and health, with her Long-haired Chihuahua, Big and shares a home with her fiancé, on whom she tests her recipes.

Together with Juan-Carlos Cruz, she is looking forward to getting people excited about food by improving the sex lives of home cooks everywhere!